Dementia Care

Dementia Care

A Care Worker Handbook

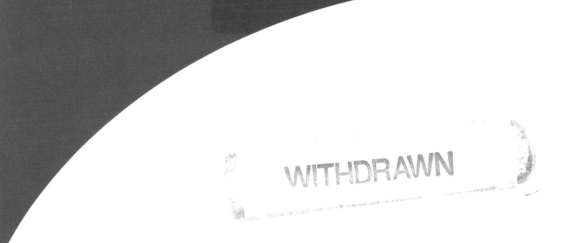

Belinda Goode and Gayle Booth

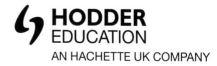

**HODDER
EDUCATION**

AN HACHETTE UK COMPANY

Orders: please contact Bookpoint Ltd, 130 Milton Park, Abingdon, Oxon
OX14 4SB. Telephone: (44) 01235 827720. Fax: (44) 01235 400454. Lines are
open from 9.00–5.00, Monday to Saturday, with a 24 hour message
answering service. You can also order through our website
www.hoddereducation.co.uk

If you have any comments to make about this, or any of our other titles,
please send them to educationenquiries@hodder.co.uk

British Library Cataloguing in Publication Data
A catalogue record for this title is available from the British Library

ISBN: 978 1 444 16322 3

First Edition Published 2012
Impression number   10 9 8 7 6 5 4 3 2 1
Year   2015 2014 2013 2012

Hachette UK's policy is to use papers that are natural, renewable and
recyclable products and made from wood grown in sustainable forests.
The logging and manufacturing processes are expected to conform to the
environmental regulations of the country of origin.

Cover photo © Alexander Raths.
Illustrations by Barking Dog Art.
Typeset by Pantek Media, Maidstone, Kent.
Printed in Italy for Hodder Education, An Hachette UK Company,
338 Euston Road, London NW1 3BH by LEGO

Contents

Acknowledgements

The authors would like to acknowledge the work of the Alzheimer's Society, Christine Bryden, Tom Kitwood, Naomi Feil, Tribal Group and SCIE Dementia Gateway, all of whom are referenced in this book.

Every effort has been made to trace and acknowledge ownership of copyright. The publishers will be glad to make suitable arrangements with any copyright holders whom it has not been possible to contact.

Photo credits

Figure 1.1 © Suprijono Suharjoto – Fotolia.com; Figure 1.3 © picsfive – Fotolia.com; Figure 1.4 © Crown Copyright; Figure 2.1 © Monkey Business – Fotolia.com; Figure 2.7 © Werner Otto/Alamy; Figure 31 © Brebca – Fotolia.com; Figure 3.9 © Rido – Fotolia.com; Figure 4.1 © Eric Isselée – Fotolia.com; Figure 4.2 © Golden Pixels LLC/Alamy; Figure 4.3 © Alistair Berg/Getty Images; Figure 4.5 © Queerstock, Inc./Alamy; Figure 5.2 © nyul – Fotolia.com; Figure 5.3 © irina86roibu – Fotolia.com; Figure 5.4 © WavebreakmediaMicro – Fotolia.com; Figure 5.5 © INTERFOTO/Alamy; Figure 5.8 © Lisa F. Young – Fotolia.com; Figure 6.1 © DIA – Fotolia.com; Figure 6.2 © nsphotography – Fotolia.com; Figure 6.3 © forestpath – Fotolia.com; Figure 6.4 © evanto/Alamy; Figure 6.5 © alexskopje – Fotolia.com; Figure 6.8 © Blend Images/Alamy; Figure 7.1 © shadowvincent – Fotolia.com; Figure 7.3 © Crown Copyright; Figure 7.6 © Monkey Business – Fotolia.com.

Walkthrough

We want you to succeed!

This book has been designed to include all the topic knowledge, assessment support and practical advice you will need for the following qualifications.

- Level 2 Award or Certificate in Awareness of Dementia
- Level 3 Award or Certificate in Awareness of Dementia
- Level 2 Diploma Health and Social Care Dementia Pathway
- Level 3 Diploma Health and Social Care Dementia Pathway.

The book has been written with the work-based learner in mind. Everything in it reflects the assessment criteria and evidence based approach that is applied to this vocational qualification.

In the pages that follow you will find up-to-date resource material which will develop your knowledge, rehearse your skills and help you to gain your qualification.

Prepare for what you are going to cover in this unit, and prepare for assessment:

The reading and activities in this unit will help you to:

- Understand what dementia is
- Understand key features of the theoretical models of dementia
- Know the most common types of dementia and their causes
- Understand factors relating to an individual's experience of dementia

Reinforce concepts with hands-on learning and generate evidence for assignments

Time to reflect

(3.1) Know the most common types of dementia and their causes

Reflect on what you have heard other people, including the media, assume about 'dementia'. Do you think this is accurate – and if not, what can you do to help the people you know understand more about dementia?

Reinforce concepts with hands-on learning and generate evidence for assignments

Evidence activity

 1.1 Communication context

Describe a situation when the context of a situation caused you to communicate in a particular non-verbal way.

Research and investigate

3.1 Care planning

Look at some care plans in the area you work. How well do they reflect the communication strengths, needs and preferences of the people you support? How could you improve the care plan?

Understand how your learning fits into real life and your working environment

Case Study

2.1 Mr Jones

Mr Jones attends a day centre. He used to be a waiter and is constantly following a care assistant about. She is becoming irritated with him, and feels that he is just pestering her. Using a person centred approach, her colleague talks to Mr Jones and listens to his stories about being a waiter. She decides to take action to improve his situation at the day centre. Using the principles of inclusion and valuing people by engaging them in everyday life, what do you think the new person centred approach would include?)

Check new words and what they mean

Key terms

Aphasia is an acquired communication disorder that impairs a person's ability to process language, but does not affect intelligence.
www.aphasia.org
Agnosia is an inability to recognise objects, faces or surroundings.

You've just covered a whole unit so here's a guide to what assessors will be looking for and links to activities that can help impress them

Assessment Summary DEM 207

Your reading of this unit and completion of the activities will have prepared you to care for or give support to individuals with dementia in a wide range of settings. The unit introduces the concepts of equality, diversity and inclusion that are fundamental to person centred care practice.

To achieve the unit, your assessor will require you to:

Learning Outcomes	Assessment Criteria
1 Understand and appreciate the importance of diversity of individuals with dementia	**1.1** Explain the importance of recognising that individuals with dementia have unique needs and preferences **See evidence activity 1.1, page 97**
	1.2 Describe ways of helping carers and others to understand that an individual with dementia has unique needs and preference **See evidence activity 1.2, page 98**
2 Understand the importance of person centred approaches in the care and support of individuals with dementia	**2.1** Describe how an individual may feel valued, included and able to engage in daily life **See case study 2.1, page 99**
	2.2 Describe how individuals with dementia may feel excluded **See case study 2.2, page 100**

Awareness and Understanding of Dementia

DEM 201 Dementia awareness

What are you finding out?

In this unit you will learn about the main causes, types and effects of dementia. We will look at the signs and symptoms and examine the attitude of society to dementia. We will go on to understand the experience of dementia. Dementia is not a disease, rather it is the term used to describe the symptoms caused by certain diseases or conditions of the brain. These symptoms involve a progressive decline in a person's abilities. In this section we will understand what is meant by the term 'dementia', and the key features of the theories of dementia. We will go on to look at the most common types of dementia and their causes and how dementia affects the individual.

The reading and activities in this unit will help you to:

• Understand what dementia is

• Understand key features of the theoretical models of dementia

• Know the most common types of dementia and their causes

• Understand factors relating to an individual's experience of dementia

LO1 Understand what dementia is

1.1 What is meant by the term 'dementia'?

The brain is part of the nervous system of the body, a network of nerve cells carrying 'messages' to different parts of the body. We will look at this in more detail in the next unit (DEM 301, p.13).

The brain has billions of nerve cells with many projections called 'dendrites'. These connect nerve cells and at the point they connect a 'synapse' is formed.

Messages travel in tiny electrical impulses and when one reaches the end of the dendrite it releases a neurotransmitter, which is a chemical that transmits the messages. The brain constantly passes messages and this is how it controls the things we do, for example, movement, speech and breathing.

When a disease or condition prevents nerve cells from working, they will die. Dementia is caused by the death of nerve cells in the brain. These cannot be replaced which means that dementia is a progressive disease – it gets worse over time and cannot be reversed. Dementia is also described as a 'long term condition' because it takes months and years to progress and as yet there is no actual cure. It is a degenerative condition and is **indiscriminate**.

Key terms

Indiscriminate means showing no distinction between race, social background or geographical location.

Dementia is not a natural part of ageing, although the chances of developing dementia increase with age. People in their mid-life can be affected. People in their 30s have been diagnosed with dementia.

It is estimated that there are currently 820,000 people diagnosed with dementia in the UK (Alzheimer's Research Trust 2010), and this will rise to over one million by 2025.

Common symptoms of dementia include:

- Memory loss (particularly short-term memory).
- Disorientation. People with dementia become more confused about time, place and person.
- Impaired cognitive abilities – difficulties with language, thinking, judgement and perception.
- Changes in behaviour. People can become withdrawn, or suspicious or agitated.
- Lack of physical coordination, the ability to sequence things (put things in the right order).

The symptoms will vary depending on the type of dementia the person experiences. It is important to remember that each person's experience of dementia is unique to them.

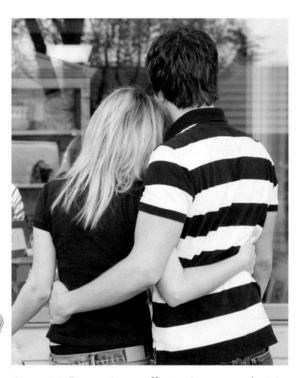

Figure 1.1 Dementia can affect younger people. It is not an inevitable part of ageing.

Evidence activity

1.1 Understand what dementia is

We have looked briefly at the common symptoms of dementia. What emotions do you think a person will feel when they are first diagnosed?

How can:

- We as care workers support them?
- Family and friends help?

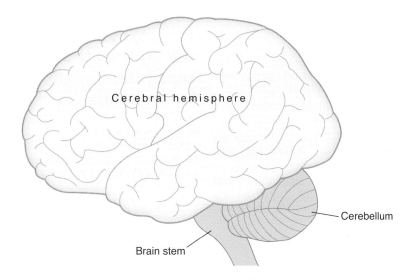

Figure 1.2

Key functions of the brain that are affected by dementia

Impaired cognitive abilities

- remembering
- communicating (we will look at this in more detail in Chapter 3, DEM 205, DEM 210, DEM 308 and DEM 312)
- understanding
- thinking
- learning
- reasoning
- planning
- evaluating.

The last four cognitive abilities are called 'executive functions'.

The loss of memory is the most common feature of dementia, and is one of its most disabling features. This is because we rely on memory to help us with most of the things we do. The person with dementia will probably find that their short-term memory is affected first.

The memory is able to work in various ways:

- It can **record** information – for example, a new name or idea.
- It can **store and retrieve** this information, so you can find it later (a bit like a filing cabinet or memory stick).

We therefore rely on our memory to learn and retain new things. This is very difficult for the person with dementia because the part of the brain responsible for learning and interpreting new information is affected by their dementia. As new learning is affected first, so the person with dementia will come to rely on their long-term memory which is damaged at a later stage of the dementia. This is why, for example, a person with dementia may not be able to remember what they ate for lunch, but they can tell you the name of their school from 50 years ago.

The human brain has three main sections.

Evidence activity

1.2 Key functions of the brain that are affected by dementia

Describe how a person with dementia might cope with short term memory loss.

The cerebral hemisphere:

- The outer layer is the cerebral cortex which helps to **control emotion thought and planning**.
- The **left side** is concerned with **speech and language, mathematical ability and logic**.
- The **right side** affects **spatial ability, face recognition, colour, shape, creativity and imagination**.

Different areas of the cerebral hemispheres have different functions:

- **The motor area** helps to control **movement**.
- **The sensory area** receives nervous impulses from sense organs in the skin and **processes them so we can feel heat, cold, touch and pain**.

- **The visual area** receives nervous impulses from the **eyes and processes them into the images that we see.**
- **The auditory area** receives nervous impulses from the **ears and processes them into the sounds we hear.**
- The **cerebellum** controls **movement, posture and coordination.**
- **The brain stem** controls vital living functions like **breathing, heartbeat and blood pressure.**
- **The limbic system** contains the **hippocampus** and is in the centre of the brain. The hippocampus controls emotions, memories and new learning.

Summary of the effects of dementia on the brain

- Parietal Lobe – Affects language, reading, writing, judging distance and sequencing.
- Frontal Lobe – Difficulty in planning and interpreting the world around us.
- Temporal Lobe – Affects verbal memory (names, etc.) and visual (forgetting who people are).
- Cerebellum – Affects balance and coordination.
- Occipital Lobe – Affects how we see things.

Case Study

 Mr Brown

Mr Brown attends the day centre each week. He loves to play dominoes and cards. You begin to notice that he is struggling to put the dominoes out in the right order and forgets which card to play next. He has recently been diagnosed with dementia.

Which part of his brain do you think has been affected?

How can you support Mr Brown?

1.3 Why depression, delirium and age-related memory impairment might be mistaken for dementia

Depression

Depression is a common symptom of dementia, but the two are not the same. People with or without dementia can suffer from depression. We can all feel 'blue' or fed up at times – this is normal because we usually feel better after a time. Depression is different. It is characterised by feelings of hopelessness that do not go away. People can have low self-esteem, and feelings of guilt and sadness as well as thoughts of self-harm and death. Depression can make people agitated, and anxious. They may sleep too much or be wakeful at night. They often lose interest in the world around them. One significant symptom of depression is forgetfulness or an inability to concentrate. People can become pre-occupied with negative thoughts. These symptoms can therefore be confused with those of dementia. The onset of depression is gradual (over weeks or months). Depression must be taken seriously at all times and if you are concerned that someone appears to have the symptoms you must seek advice and support for them.

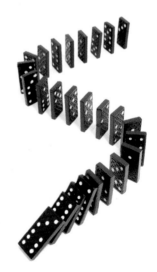

Figure 1.3 Dementia affects different aspects of functioning, leading to further problems in communication, sequencing and so on.

Delirium

The symptoms of delirium are very similar to those of dementia. Like depression, people with dementia can get delirium, and in fact people with dementia who are ill are more at risk of having delirium. The main symptoms of delirium are fluctuating alertness, changes in sleep pattern, disorganised thoughts and illusions and delusions. People can be agitated or withdrawn. They have difficulty concentrating and can be very emotional. Unlike dementia the onset is sudden, either hours or days. Again, it is very important to be observant when a person with dementia is ill, particularly if they have contracted an infection, or are taking more than four types of medication (**polypharmacy**).These are some of the main causes of delirium and, as the onset is sudden, any changes in the person should be immediately assessed and treated.

Memory impairment

We all have difficulty remembering things to a greater or lesser extent. As we get older this is more likely to increase and it is natural for people to assume they are developing a dementia type illness. Some memory loss can be caused by medication, depression, and physical illnesses like diabetes or pernicious anaemia. However, for most of us this will be a normal part of the ageing process. This age-related memory impairment is sometimes called 'mild cognitive impairment' and there are theories that a healthy diet, exercise and 'brain training' can help slow the onset.

It is only when memory loss begins to stop a person from carrying out normal activities of daily living that they should seek advice and treatment.

Evidence activity

 Why depression, delirium and age-related memory impairment might be mistaken for dementia

Complete a table that demonstrates your understanding of the main symptoms of dementia, delirium, memory loss and depression.

LO2 Understand the key features of the theoretical models of dementia

 Key terms

'Model' is a tool that explains a theory to make it more understandable.

2.1 The medical model of dementia

The 'medical model' of dementia takes physical impairments to be of primary concern, and, more broadly, considers physical impairments to be barriers to society. Therefore the medical model of dementia takes the progressive cognitive and physical decline in individuals with dementia as being the reason why they cannot carry out everyday tasks.

This is the model that was widely used in the West until the 1990s. The medical model views dementia as an organic brain disorder that causes impaired cognitive abilities. Because it is viewed primarily as a 'disease', it is seen as a problem that can only be dealt with by medical experts. The 'patient' who 'suffers' from dementia must be treated and cared for. This view sees the disease in control of the person, and does not particularly take into account all the other elements in the life of the person with dementia. It is not a person centred or holistic model. There are still some professionals who view dementia in this way. People with dementia have reported instances when they were told it was a normal part of ageing and their symptoms have been dismissed. There is still a common misconception that 'nothing can be done' and if this is the case 'what is the point of diagnosing dementia?'. This results in people being reluctant to visit their GP or feeling stigmatised because they may have this 'illness'. Unfortunately, this can mean that assessment and treatment come much later in the dementia journey, often when a crisis occurs.

2.2 The social model of dementia

The 'social model' of disability considers the social context of barriers that may prevent or inhibit a person's ability to participate and is primarily concerned with the concept of disabilities and needs. It is focused on aspects of the disease that can be adapted or managed in a particular way that in some ways could be viewed as maintaining or rehabilitation.

The National Dementia Strategy 2009 (Department of Health) strongly supports the social model of dementia. It talks about 'living well with dementia'.

The social model does not see the person with the illness or disease as the problem; rather it sees society as the problem. The negative way society views dementia and people who live with dementia can make it difficult for them to access diagnosis, treatment and support. The social model emphasises that we must see the person first, that we should understand the experience of the person with dementia and by doing so society should ensure people are able to access person centred services and support.

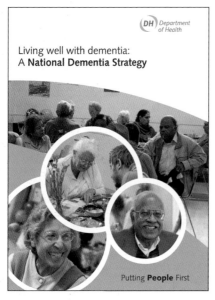

Figure 1.4 The objectives of the National Dementia Strategy 2009 emphasise how we must as a society promote 'living well with dementia'.

  Research and investigate

2.1 2.2 Models of dementia

Look around your workplace and the surrounding neighbourhood for barriers that prevent people with particular needs from living as normal and fulfilling a life as possible. What does this tell you about some of society's attitudes to people with a disability?

 ## Dementia as a disability

The medical model tends to see a disability as a limitation. It concentrates on what the person cannot do rather than what is still possible for them. The social model of disability arose because people with disabilities rejected this idea and the effect it was having on their lives. They argued that labels like 'disabled' or 'limited' not only stigmatised them but also did not take into account their personhood, skills and abilities. Labels are also barriers to some parts of society like housing, social events, transport and education. If venues like concert halls, museums, or shops, universities and so on are adapted to ensure access for wheelchair users they are not limited.

Researchers have conducted numerous studies that have found that despite dementia being a medical and physical condition it actually causes excess disability through a lack of understanding of key issues. Put simply – underestimating the significance of the physical and social environment can lead to the manufacture of disability.

Research and investigate

2.3 Dementia as a disability

The Disability Discrimination Act. Find out what the DDA tells us about not discriminating against a person with a disability.

LO3 Know the most common types of dementia and their causes

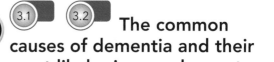 **The common causes of dementia and their most likely signs and symptoms**

There are over one hundred different types of dementia. Many people assume Alzheimer's disease is the only name for the condition.

Time to reflect

3.1 Know the most common types of dementia and their causes

Reflect on what you have heard other people, including the media, assume about 'dementia'. Do you think this is accurate – and if not, what can you do to help the people you know understand more about dementia?

The following explanations are of the most common types of dementia.

Alzheimer's disease (AD)

This is the most common cause of dementia and represents around 60 per cent of all cases. It is characterised by amyloid '**plaques**' and neurofibral '**tangles**' in brain structures that lead to the death of brain cells. It is progressive, affecting more parts of the brain over time.

Key terms

Plaques are insoluble protein deposits that build up around nerve cells.

Tangles are insoluble twisted protein fibres that build up inside nerve cells.

There is also a general loss of brain cells and a significant shrinkage in brain tissue. AD is usually slow and gradual.

Signs and symptoms

It affects the ability to remember, speak and think clearly and rationally.

In the early stages the person may be mildly forgetful; they may have problems finding the right words and lose interest in hobbies etc.

As the disease progresses (moderate stage) memory loss and 'word finding' become worse. The person may be confused by new surroundings and have trouble recognising familiar people and places. They find difficulty undertaking everyday tasks.

In the later (advanced stage) the person becomes completely dependent on others, has difficulty eating and walking, controlling bodily functions and understanding their environment.

Vascular dementia (VaD)

Represents around 15–20 per cent of all cases and is the second most common type of dementia. It is caused by blockages in blood supply to the brain. The lack of blood and oxygen supply to nerve cells means they die. Areas of the brain damaged this way are called 'infarcts'. Vascular dementia is sometimes called 'multi-infarct dementia' and is due to a series of strokes.

Signs and symptoms

People with vascular dementia have symptoms similar to other dementias but in particular they have problems concentrating and communicating. There may be a 'step-like' progression of the dementia. The person may have a stroke causing some deterioration and then a settling or plateau of symptoms followed by another dip because of a stroke. Onset is more obvious than AD. The person may become restless, more 'wandering' and struggle with memory problems and incontinence. Vascular dementia tends to affect particular areas of the brain which means the person may retain more insight into their situation and hence become depressed.

Dementia with Lewy bodies (DLB)

This is a result of small round protein deposits found in nerve cells. The protein deposits in the brain obstruct chemical messages in the brain which disrupts normal brain functions. Lewy bodies are also found in the brains of people with Parkinson's disease, and some people with Parkinson's disease will go on to develop a Lewy body type dementia.

Signs and symptoms

People with DLB usually have symptoms similar to those of AD and Parkinson's disease. They may have problems with attention, alertness and disorientation, as well as being unable to plan ahead. They may develop the symptoms of Parkinson's disease, including loss of facial expression, slowness and rigidity of limbs and changes in strength and tone of voice. DLB can be variable from day to day. Tasks that were completed yesterday may be impossible today. This is why a person with DLB can often be labelled as lazy or manipulative. Approximately 10 per cent of people with dementia have DLB.

Fronto temporal dementia (FTD)

Represents around 5 per cent of all cases and is a progressive degeneration of the frontal lobes of the brain. It includes Pick's disease. All are caused by damage to parts of the brain that are responsible for our behaviour, emotions and language.

Signs and symptoms

There will be some experience of personality and behaviour changes. The person may lose the ability to empathise with others (see things from the other person's point of view).The person may change from being introverted to being extroverted or vice versa. This means that they can become disinhibited, making tactless and rude comments. Their social skills can become blunted and they can develop particular routines or rituals. They may have language difficulties, with 'pressure of speech', using many words to describe a simple concept, or speak less and less. They are also susceptible to overeating and developing a 'sweet tooth'.

Korsakoff's syndrome (KS)

This is caused by a lack of vitamin B1 which damages the brain and nervous system and is usually associated with heavy consumption of alcohol over a long period of time. Alcohol can inflame the stomach lining, preventing the body from absorbing vitamin B1. People who drink heavily also tend to have a poor diet and so do not compensate for the lack of vitamin B1. About 2 per cent of people with dementia will have KS.

Signs and symptoms

The main symptom is memory loss, particularly those things that happened after the onset of the condition. Other symptoms include difficulty in learning new information and skills, personality changes from apathy to talkative and repetitive behaviour. The person may not realise they have the condition and will invent things to cover the gaps in their memory. This is called 'confabulation'.

Creutzfeldt-Jakob disease (CJD)

This is a type of **prion** disease. Prions are proteins that occur naturally on the surface of nerve cells in the brain but cause progressive nerve damage if they become faulty.

Signs and symptoms

There are changes in personality, depression and loss of interest in life. As the condition progresses there can be confusion, memory loss, anxiety, delusions, loss of balance, difficulty in hearing and seeing, speech loss and paralysis. CJD is quite rare.

Some people are diagnosed with a 'mixed dementia'. It is common to be diagnosed with a combination of AD and VaD.

> ### Evidence activity
>
>   **Know the most common types of dementia and their causes**
>
> Produce a leaflet for staff which explains each type of dementia, its causes and symptoms.

A word of caution...

Although it can be helpful to understand the nature and causes of the different types of dementia, it is more important to see **the person** not the condition **first**. Each person will be different and we must not make assumptions that they will behave in any particular way because they have a certain type of dementia. This is the essence of person centred care which we will talk about more in Chapter 2, DEM 202 and DEM 204.

3.3 3.4 **The risk factors and prevalence rates for the most common causes of dementia**

- Age (one third of people over 95 have dementia. The proportion of people aged 85 and over with dementia is between 25 and 35 per cent).
- Gender (about two thirds of people with dementia are women, however women have a longer life expectancy than men).
- Low level of education (education can slow down the early symptoms of dementia, educated people have been found to have less nerve damage).
- Lung and heart conditions which compromise blood and oxygen supply to the brain.
- Poisoning.
- Weak immune system.
- Repeated head injuries.
- Vitamin B deficiency.
- Unhealthy lifestyle, including heavy smoking, drinking and obesity.
- History of stroke, high blood pressure and cholesterol.
- Learning difficulties like Down's syndrome (studies have shown that people with Down's syndrome develop the plaques and tangles associated with Alzheimer's disease).
- Family history of dementia.

Other prevalence rates

Remember that these relate to people who are diagnosed with dementia. We know that there are significant numbers of people who, for many reasons, may not yet be diagnosed.

- 75 per cent of people with dementia have either Alzheimer's disease or vascular dementia or a combination of both.
- There are over 11,500 people with dementia from black or minority ethnic groups.
- There are currently between 16,000 and 25,000 people under the age of 65 with dementia in the UK.
- 60,000 deaths a year are directly attributable to dementia.
- If we delayed the onset of dementia by 5 years we could halve this number.
- Two thirds of people with dementia live in the community.
- 64 per cent of people living in care homes have a form of dementia.

  www.alzheimers.org.uk
  www.bgs.org.uk
  www.cjd.ed.ac.uk
  www.hpa.org.uk

Evidence activity

 The risk factors and prevalence rates for the most common causes of dementia

Use an internet search engine, journals and reports produced by your local health and social care providers to find out the prevalence rates for different types of dementia in your area.

LO4 Understand factors relating to an individual's experience of dementia

 Describe how different individuals may experience living with dementia depending on age, type of dementia, and level of ability and disability

 ## Research and investigate

4.1 Describe how different individuals may experience living with dementia

Think about the people you know who may have been diagnosed with dementia. What are their different experiences? What skills and personal attributes do they still have? What have they lost?

Age

The incidence of dementia increases with age. Older people with symptoms of dementia may be discriminated against because dementia is dismissed as a 'normal' part of ageing. They may therefore have difficulty accessing the right services and support. The stigma associated with ageing and dementia can mean that older people are disregarded and their views and needs are not taken seriously. It is also likely that the carer for the person with dementia is also older, or that they have to rely more heavily on grown-up sons and daughters. This can be very difficult as well. It will depend on how far the person with dementia can preserve their relationships. We will discuss this more in Unit DEM 301.

Being diagnosed with dementia at an earlier age brings with it very different problems. The older person has probably retired and does not have children who are dependent on them. This is not the case for the person under the age of 65. They are often unprepared for such a diagnosis and unless given support from the beginning can quickly feel that all hope is lost. They may still have a job and children at school. Financial and family concerns add to the pressure of the diagnosis. Because, as a society, we still associate dementia with older people there is limited public and professional awareness and understanding of younger onset dementia and this can make it difficult for younger people with dementia to find appropriate support.

Type of dementia

Most people will have heard about the main diseases or conditions that cause dementia and can perhaps empathise more with a person with Alzheimer's disease, for example, because it has had media coverage. This is possibly not the case for the more rare types of dementia or when the person with dementia begins to show a change in their personality or behaviour. They may experience some hostility, particularly if they are perceived to be difficult or challenging or aggressive.

Level of ability

A person's experience of dementia will be shaped by **external and internal factors**. Tom Kitwood talks about **internal factors** like personality and health. For example, if the person has always been confident and optimistic in their approach to life, they may find more positive ways of managing their illness. These are called 'coping strategies'.

If they have problems with their physical health, this might have a negative impact on the dementia. For example, arthritis and an inability to move about may make a further problem like dementia feel worse.

Tom Kitwood was a senior lecturer at the University of Bradford. He developed a keen interest in dementia, particularly person centred dementia care, and became the leader of the Bradford Dementia Group, which continues today.

External factors include the environment the person lives in and their wider social network. Friendships can be lost because people find it difficult to communicate with the person with dementia. Family relationships change and can become awkward as family members have to take on an increasingly caring role.

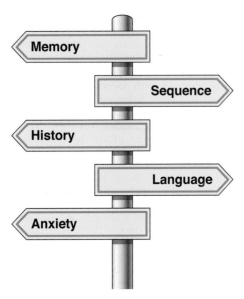

Figure 1.5 The signs that we normally rely on become confusing and less meaningful.

The physical environment is a problem as it begins to make less sense to the person with dementia.

Level of disability

The degree of damage will depend on the type of dementia and in some cases, like Alzheimer's disease, whether treatment begins in a timely way,

to slow down the progress of the condition. The person's experience of dementia may also be influenced by the way the dementia is perceived as a disability. If the person's disabilities are not compensated for by adapting their environment, or the way we communicate with them, for example, then we have emphasised the disability rather than supported the person to overcome or manage it.

4.2 Outline the impact that the attitudes and behaviours of others may have on an individual with dementia

Society and the media

'One day I hope that we will treat people with dementia with respect, recognise just how hard they are trying to cope with getting through each day, and provide them with appropriate emotional support, social networks and encouragement'.

Christine Bryden *Dancing with Dementia* 2005.

Christine Bryden was diagnosed with dementia at the age of 46. She experienced some of the prejudice associated with dementia. Unless we remove the stigma and discrimination shown towards people with dementia and support them instead, they will struggle to cope with their condition and to have their 'personhood' recognised.

Time to reflect

4.1 The impact that attitudes and behaviours of others may have

Think about how your family, friends and colleagues behave towards people with mental health conditions such as dementia. If they exhibit negative views or attitudes, why do you think this is? How could you help them in changing these views and behaviours?

The media does not always portray a positive image of living with dementia. The stereotype of the person as a 'victim' who is unable to have any control is common.

This attitude is partly due to a lack of knowledge. The more we understand about dementia, the more we can help.

The family and individuals

People cannot be experts in dementia simply because a family member develops the condition. As the person moves along their dementia journey, so will family and friends develop their knowledge and understanding. At the beginning of the journey they may feel embarrassed, frustrated and anxious. There can be a sense of 'loss' for the person they once knew. They may reflect a more general view that the person only has themselves to blame, that they should stop behaving in the way they do or pull themselves together. These attitudes can be very damaging to the person with dementia because they do not recognise the struggle the person is experiencing. As a result the person with dementia can feel isolated and lose their self-confidence and self-esteem. If their communication skills are affected they may also have problems expressing how they feel and become more excluded.

A national response

The National Dementia Strategy 2009 (Department of Health) recognised that more must be done to change the attitude and behaviours of society, as well as health and social care organisations. The strategy has seventeen objectives. The first three objectives deal with how we perceive dementia.

Objective 1: Improving public and professional awareness and understanding of dementia. This sparked a national campaign which portrayed people 'living well with dementia' and aimed to help the public understand that dementia should not be used to stigmatise people.

Objective 2: Good-quality early diagnosis and intervention for all. This encourages GPs and other medical professionals to be more vigilant when assessing people and to refer people to specialist services as soon as possible. The earlier in the condition people receive treatment, the more likely they are to have a positive outcome.

Objective 3: Good-quality information for those with diagnosed dementia and their carers. Part of the problem is fear due to a lack of knowledge.

There are many health and social care professionals supporting people with dementia and their carers. Good practice dictates that professionals and the general public become well informed about dementia and the impact it has on the people living with it. If this can be achieved then the stigma and prejudice associated with dementia can be a thing of the past.

Evidence activity

 4.2 The impact that attitudes and behaviours of others may have

Produce an information sheet for colleagues and visitors to your workplace that:

- explains the negative attitudes people can have towards dementia
- describes the impact that these attitudes can have on people living with dementia

Assessment Summary DEM 201

Reading this unit and completing the activities will have provided you with knowledge, understanding and skills required to improve your awareness of dementia.
To achieve the unit, your assessor will require you to:

Learning Outcomes	Assessment Criteria
1 Understand what dementia is	**1.1** Explain what is meant by the term "dementia" See evidence activity 1.1, page 3
	1.2 Describe the key functions of the brain that are affected by dementia See evidence activity 1.2, page 3
	1.3 Explain why depression, delirium and age-related memory impairment may be mistaken for dementia See evidence activity 1.3, page 5

Learning Outcomes	Assessment Criteria	
2 Understand the key features of the theoretical models of dementia	**2.1**	Outline the medical mode of dementia See research and investigate activity 2.1, page 6
	2.2	Outline the social model of dementia See research and investigate activity 2.2, page 6
	2.3	Explain why dementia should be seen as a disability See research and investigate activity 2.3, page 6
3 Know the most common types of dementia and their causes	**3.1**	List the most common causes of dementia See evidence activity 3.1, page 8
	3.2	Describe the likely signs and symptoms of the most common causes of dementia See evidence activity 3.2, page 8
	3.3	Outline the risk factors for the most common causes of dementia See evidence activity 3.3, page 9
	3.4	Identify prevalence rates for different types of dementia See evidence activity 3.4, page 9
4 Understand factors relating to an individual's experience of dementia	**4.1**	Describe how different individuals may experience living with dementia depending on age, type of dementia, and level of ability and disability See research and investigate activity 4.1, page 9
	4.2	Outline the impact that attitudes and behaviours of others may have on an individual with dementia See evidence activity 4.2, page 11

DEM 301 Understand the process and experience of dementia

What are you finding out?

We learnt in the first unit that dementia is not a specific disease. It is an 'umbrella' term for a collection of symptoms caused by a number of disorders that affect the brain. Dementia is a common condition that currently affects over 800,000 people in the UK. Dementia costs the UK economy around £23 billion a year, more than cancer and heart disease combined.

People with dementia have damaged **cognitive functioning** that interferes with activities of daily living. They lose their ability to solve problems and learn. They may find it difficult to control their emotions and experience some personality changes. Symptoms also include agitation, delusions and hallucinations. Memory loss is a common symptom of dementia but on its own does not indicate a diagnosis of the condition. Specialist tests must be carried out and more in-depth assessment of the person done before a diagnosis can be made.

There are also physical changes, because of the brain's difficulties in sending messages for swallowing or sequential movements.

Key terms

Cognitive functioning is difficulty in carrying out intellectual functions, such as learning, thinking and remembering.

Reading this unit and carrying out the activities will enable you to:

- Understand the neurology of dementia
- Understand the impact of recognition and diagnosis of dementia
- Understand how dementia care must be underpinned by a person centred approach

LO1 Understand the neurology of dementia

1.1 Describe a range of causes of dementia syndrome

We will begin by looking at how the brain works and how different conditions affect the function of the brain.

The brain consists of three main sections:

- **The hindbrain** – mainly concerned with basic life support functions.
- **The midbrain.**
- **The forebrain** – commands the majority of the higher brain functions, such as memory and language.

To assist our understanding of the different parts of the brain, the forebrain has been divided up into four '**lobes**', shown in Figure 1.6.

The **occipital lobe** is located at the back of the brain and deals primarily with information that is passed from the eyes. The eyes convert sensory information about light which is interpreted by the brain. As there are two stages to being able to interpret visual stimuli, we need to think about the eye and the brain working together to see things. The ability to see is accomplished by the eye. What follows is perception which is interpreted by the occipital and parietal lobes. These lobes interpret information about colour, shape and movement.

Even if a person with dementia has perfectly good eyesight, problems with the occipital and parietal lobes could mean they have difficulty in perceiving and seeing things. It is important that a person with dementia who has difficulty with their sight wears suitable glasses and has regular eye examinations so that the brain can gather and utilise as much information as possible.

The **parietal lobe** processes information about where objects are located around them, how information is perceived, the significance of situations and the sequence of putting things together.

The dominant parietal lobe (usually the left half) is concerned with the things we put together in sequence or order. For example, tasks such as reading, writing and maths are commanded by our dominant parietal lobe.

This side of the parietal lobe is involved in a condition known as **apraxia**, an impairment of learned purposive movements. A common example of this is 'Dressing apraxia' in people living with **Alzheimer's disease**, which results in forgetting co-ordination and the movements needed to dress oneself so that for example the order of clothes and the ability to fasten a belt could be impaired.

Our dominant parietal lobe also tells us our left from our right, and makes us aware of where our limbs are when we are doing things. For example, when the dominant parietal lobe makes sure that our arm is far enough away from our body when pouring the kettle while we are making a cup of tea.

The non-dominant parietal lobe receives information from the eyes from the occipital lobe. The function of this area is to combine spatial information with basic sensory information about colour, perception and size. When this area of the brain is damaged it can lead to symptoms known as '**visual agnosia**' or **visual perceptual difficulties**. Put simply, this is a difficulty in recognising objects, faces or surroundings.

The **temporal lobe** lies beneath the parietal lobe and is involved in processing memory and language.

The **frontal lobe** is made up of parts which work together to form our 'executive' or 'management' centre. These parts carry out the following activities:

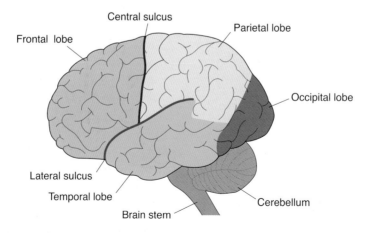

Figure 1.6 How each area of the brain controls different areas of function.

- **Planning actions and learning new tasks** – The outer layers of the front part of the brain are important for organising and planning what we do and our ability to learn new things. For someone who has damage in this area of the brain many everyday activities which comprise of multi-stage elements can be difficult. For example, a task such as shopping, which would involve compiling a shopping list, going to the shops, identifying the items needed and orientation around the supermarket, can become difficult. This is because the different stages and timings of the ways in which we would do these have been affected by the damage to this area of the brain.

- **Motivation** – In between the two hemispheres of the brain, the middle portion of the frontal lobe creates motivation. If this part of the brain is damaged people may become sluggish, so that for example they might not want to get out of bed or to become involved in activities. It is important not to assume that the person is being lazy but instead remember that it might be because this area of the brain is damaged.

- **Dis-inhibition** – The way we behave in relation to the different social contexts that we frequent has been found to be commanded by the frontal lobe. When our brain is working properly, this part of the brain provides us with information that moderates our behaviour. It tells us when not to swear at someone even when they are being unacceptable towards us. For people living with dementia this area of the brain could be damaged, which can lead to behaviour we might find socially unacceptable. Therefore it is important for us to understand that it is the damage caused by the condition, not the person, and to remember the person with dementia does not really mean to say or behave in an unacceptable way.

The hemispheres

In addition to being divided into lobes, the brain is also physically divided into two hemispheres. By this we mean the brain is split into left and right sides. It is essential to remember that the different parts to the brain are not completely separate because they are joined by structures that mean they can communicate and share information with one another.

Diseases and conditions that cause dementia

- **Alzheimer's disease** is characterised by amyloid '**plaques**' and '**tangles**' in brain structures that lead to the death of brain cells. It is progressive and over time affects more parts and areas of the brain. As a result of the loss of cells shrinkage of the brain structure occurs.

- **Vascular dementia** is caused by blockages in blood supply to the brain. The lack of blood and oxygen supply to nerve cells means they die. Areas of the brain damaged this way are called '**infarcts**'.

- **Dementia with Lewy bodies** is when protein deposits in the brain obstruct chemical messages in the brain which disrupts normal brain functions

- **Fronto-temporal dementia** is a progressive degeneration of the frontal lobes of the brain. It includes Pick's disease. All are caused by damage to parts of the brain that are responsible for our behaviour, emotions and language.

- Some people are diagnosed with a mixed dementia, commonly Alzheimer's disease and vascular dementia.

Research into the causes and possible cure for dementia is now more prominent in the media. These are some examples from Alzheimer's Research UK and the Alzheimer's Society.

In 2008 Sir Terry Pratchett donated $1million to the Alzheimer's Research Trust and became a patron. He has been diagnosed with a rare form of Alzheimer's disease. He said: 'I'd eat the arse out of a dead mole if it offered a fighting chance'.

In 2009 the Alzheimer's Research Trust scientists discovered two new genes related to Alzheimer's disease.

In 2010 a University of Oxford project funded by the Alzheimer's Research Trust found that daily tablets of B vitamins can halve the rate of brain shrinkage in elderly people with mild cognitive impairment (MCI).

Currently the Alzheimer's Society research projects are investigating how changes in Alzheimer's disease affects the balance of iron in brain cells. They are also mapping differences in mental ability between people with and without dementia

Evidence activity

 Describe a range of causes of dementia

Create a table explaining the different parts of the brain, what they do and how dementia in its various forms impacts on the functions of the brain.

Write three case studies about people with dementia, in which you describe the condition. Describe three types of dementia, and remember to respect confidentiality.

1.2 Describe the types of memory impairment commonly experienced by individuals with dementia

Memory is the ability to **store**, **retain** and **recall** information. We have learnt that memory problems are usually the first and most obvious symptom that will present in people with dementia. In most cases, short term memory is affected, with the most recent events being the first to be forgotten. For example, a person with early stages of dementia might simply forget how to complete a job or activity that they began, or they may misplace objects and not know where or how to find them. However, long term memories are much easier to recall even when dementia is in latter stages. Many people with dementia can still recall and talk about their childhood and early life. As dementia progresses, the capacity of the brain to store and recall information of recent events becomes so affected that the person loses a sense of the present and the remembered past becomes their reality.

The areas of the brain that process the way we use our memory when we understand visual information can affect people's ability to recall words. This means that verbal impairment is commonly experienced by people living with dementia.

Although we know a lot about the brain, we still do not know specifically where our long-term memories are stored. It seems that earlier recollections, like family life, school days and work, are located in long term memory. This may be significant as events may have been rehearsed, recited and revisited more than short term memories about today or last week. This could be why a person living with dementia may be able to discuss their childhood events much more easily than recalling an activity that they have just completed.

In summary, the memory is responsible for:

- storing new information
- remembering and recalling recent events
- remembering and recalling places and people.

Evidence activity

 1.2 Describe the types of memory impairment commonly experienced

Think about some of the people you have worked with or know. What signs of memory loss did they show? What was their reaction to this? What was the reaction of the people around them?

1.3 Explain the way that individuals process information with reference to the abilities and limitations of individuals with dementia

Dementia is associated with the decline of the brain's capacity to process information. This decline can have profound effects on a person's ability to carry out daily activities, communicate, make sense of the world and make judgements.

Day to day activities where problems may occur include:

- Putting letters, words and sentences together in order to read and write.
- Combining numbers to make calculations.
- Coordinating movements, for example dressing, using implements, walking.
- Locating objects within a space, for example reaching for something.
- Thinking, planning and learning new tasks – the ability to perform tasks such as shopping and cooking get lost and cannot be retrieved. The person can also get stuck on what they are doing or saying. This is called perseveration.
- Performing particular activities because of lack of motivation (apathy).
- Problems with the '**communication cycle**'. Inability to use the correct word may lead the person to find it hard to respond as well as to understand the message.
- Problems with the visual system which causes people to misinterpret images.
- **Misperceptions** – this is when the person misinterprets pictures and so on. For example, mistaking patterns on the carpet for holes.
- **Misidentifications** – when the person cannot perceive the difference between people, for example mistaking their son for their husband.
- **Misnaming** what is seen.
- Other visual difficulties include being unable to perceive depth, contrast between colours and recognising objects.
- **A failure of insight and judgement** – not perceiving risk and danger. This leaves a person with dementia vulnerable to exploitation, as well as losing money, leaving the gas on or a lack of road sense. They may also not realise they are neglecting their personal hygiene, putting their health and dignity at risk.
- **Losing a sense of time**. Finding it hard to anticipate what is happening next.

Case Study

1.3 Mrs Green

Mrs Green is 92. She has Alzheimer's disease and lives in a care home. She is unable to make informed decisions about the major issues in her life. She is able to eat independently and go to the toilet unassisted. She cannot dress or bathe herself and is having difficulty walking independently. She is unable to verbalise her thoughts and is unaware of time. She misinterprets what she sees, and often mistakes a particular male carer for her son.

1) What reasons can you give for Mrs Green's decline in abilities?
2) What can you do to support her?
3) Write a care plan explaining that support.

1.4 Explain how other factors can cause changes in an individual's condition that may not be attributable to dementia

There are many factors other than dementia that can cause some of the problems described.

- Communication problems can be caused by a stroke or poor hearing or sight (sensory issues).
- Visual problems are often attributable to the normal ageing process, although the person who does not have dementia is usually able to adjust and compensate more for these deficits.
- Hallucinations are a common symptom of other mental health problems.
- People with dementia can experience mood swings and become agitated. This is not peculiar to dementia. Medication, drugs, alcohol, the frustrations associated with ageing, disability and poor health can also be a cause. This is also true of social problems like poor housing, a lack of support networks, having to change or compromise your lifestyle – for example, going into a care home.

- People with dementia can have problems with eating, but this can also occur when chewing and swallowing is painful, if people are depressed, or have had a stroke and have difficulty swallowing.
- Infections – can cause delirium , which has a similar presentation to dementia, but is a temporary condition if treated properly.
- Severe constipation. Can make the person confused and may even affect mobility.
- Depression. The person may become withdrawn and unresponsive to social stimulation. They may appear vague and forgetful because they have difficulty in engaging.
- Taking medication incorrectly, or taking too many medications (more than four different medications, which is called polypharmacy, can cause confusion).
- Vitamin and thyroid deficiencies.
- Brain tumours or a 'catastrophic' brain injury.

Evidence activity

1.4 How other factors can cause changes in an individual's condition

Think back to Mrs Green. Had you not known that she had been diagnosed with Alzheimer's disease, what would you attribute her limitations to? What other factors could be the cause of her problems?

1.5 Explain why the abilities and needs of an individual with dementia may fluctuate

We have already learnt that each person's experience of dementia is unique, depending on their personal history, their personality, the support they receive and their emotional resilience. Factors that influence this variation in the experience of dementia include:

- Memory – this can vary depending on how well the person may feel on a particular day, or how effective other people's communication skills are.
- Health – this may vary depending on medication taken, infections, a high temperature, constipation, pain control (or lack of it).

- Cognitive abilities – people can move between drowsiness to periods of agitation. This is the case for DLB where there are marked contrasts between being fully alert and talkative and drowsiness.
- Sleep – there may be difficulty sleeping, sleep patterns are affected and day can become night. People can be more restless at particular times of the day, for example late afternoon/early evening. This is sometimes called 'sundowning'.

We know that people with dementia are not only affected by internal factors like their health, but that their needs and abilities are influenced by the environment they live in and the way others treat them. We will consider more about the 'social model of disability' later. This model explains how we can either help or disable a person by the environment we expect them to cope with. For example, a person with dementia living in a care home that takes care to ensure there is clear signage and effective use of colours in the table layout will probably manage better than the person who is expected to live in a home with inadequate signage and a confusing use of colours and patterns.

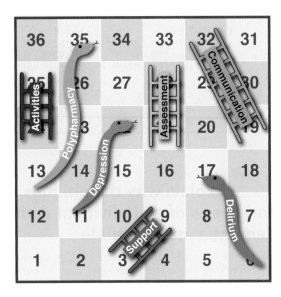

Figure 1.7 People with dementia may become more unwell if they are depressed or have a delirium, but can improve if they are given the right support in a timely way.

Time to reflect

1.5 Why the abilities and needs of an individual with dementia may fluctuate

Think about people with dementia who you know or work with. Consider why their abilities and needs may fluctuate. Look at the environment they live in – does this present them with challenges? Observe how others interact with them, is this having a particular effect? Does the person experience particular health problems which may be an issue?

LO2 Understand the impact of recognition and diagnosis of dementia

2.1 Describe the impact of early diagnosis and follow up to diagnosis

To be informed that you have a type of dementia is obviously challenging and potentially traumatic because it is a life changing condition. It also has significant implications for both the person with dementia and their family. There continues to be a stigma attached to dementia, which makes both receiving a diagnosis and living with the condition more difficult.

Evidence activity

2.1 Describe the impact of early diagnosis and follow up to diagnosis

'We had gone to him (the GP) for a lot of things and he was telling (the person with dementia) that it was in his mind, he hadn't got these problems, he needed to pull himself together'.

(Carer) Living Well with Dementia, The National Dementia strategy 2009

What attitude is being shown here by the GP? Why do you think these attitudes are still common? What is your response to these attitudes?

Diagnosis can be a relief for some people because it explains their worrying symptoms and gives the person and their family the chance to plan for the future. This is why early diagnosis is so important. If the person is diagnosed with Alzheimer's disease they may be able to begin taking anti-dementia medication which can delay the effects of dementia.

In the early stages of any dementia there is the opportunity to work out coping strategies and make decisions about the future (**advanced wishes**). Healthcare professionals should make time available to discuss the diagnosis and its implications with the person with dementia and their family (usually only with the consent of the person with dementia). Depending on the type of dementia, the reaction of the person diagnosed and family and carer dynamics, it may be necessary to offer on-going support.

In many areas of the country mental health services operate memory clinics. This service is often part of a 'pathway'. This is a person centred approach which not only assesses and diagnoses the person with dementia, but also offers post diagnostic support and education. The service might also 'signpost' people to other support networks like the local Alzheimer's society or social services, depending on the need of the person and their family.

It is extremely important that the person with dementia and their carers are supported by:

- peer and support groups
- specialist advisers
- maintaining their social networks
- being encouraged to 'live well with dementia' by living as normal a life as possible
- carer respite and education.

Research and investigate

(2.1) Describe the impact of early diagnosis and follow up to diagnosis

Use a search engine to find out more about advanced wishes. You can go to the Alzheimer's website for more information.

Time to reflect

(2.1) Describe the impact of early diagnosis and follow up to diagnosis

Why do you think it is so important for people with dementia and their carers to have as much information and support as possible?

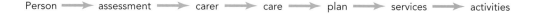
Person → assessment → carer → care → plan → services → activities

Figure 1.8 A pathway describing how the assessment, diagnosis, treatment and support of a person with dementia can be mapped out and planned as a process.

2.2 Explain the importance of recording possible signs or symptoms of dementia in an individual in line with agreed ways of working

We have learnt that the signs and symptoms of dementia can often present in a similar way to other mental health problems. It is important to understand the differences in the presentations of delirium and depression, for example. Dementia does not occur in a matter of weeks, so any acute onset of confusion may be due to other factors like infection or medication.

If you suspect a person is developing dementia, it is important to talk to them in the very early stages. It can be a very frightening experience to begin to lose some cognitive functioning like short-term memory and it is common for people to deny the problem or hide it. The person needs to know that you are not judging them or watching them in a critical way, but rather that you can offer support by listening and working with them. It is very easy to want to 'take over' very early on and this is both demeaning and probably unnecessary. Remember the principles of person centred care and put the person with suspected dementia at the centre of what you do.

When you are assessing a person you should take into account symptoms like forgetfulness, disorganised thoughts or behaviour, depression (low mood) and change in personality. This will build a picture of the problems encountered by the person. Think about:

- When the problems began.
- What functions have been affected.
- What sort of things the person forgets.
- Whether they seem low in mood – are they reluctant to talk, or disinterested in the world around them?
- Whether the person has any medical problems – what is their medical history?
- Is there a family history of dementia?
- Have you identified any risks, for example, do they leave the cooker on or forget what they were doing yesterday?
- How intense and frequent the symptoms are.
- Whether there are changes in the way the person presents or whether their needs have changed.

Your assessment can enable the GP or other professionals to gain a fuller picture of the person, and in doing so they will be able to make a more informed decision about whether it is necessary to refer the person on to secondary mental health services for an in-depth assessment.

It is also important to involve the family and carers of the person as they will be able to give you a different perspective. Most importantly, never exclude the person themselves.

Case Study

2.2 Mrs White

Mrs White was admitted to hospital from home, and seen by the hospital mental health team because she seemed confused and anxious. The family were consulted and agreed that she had also been confused at home.

What other information do you think the hospital team would ask the family for and what kind of observations would they make when assessing Mrs White's mental health needs?

2.3 Explain the process of reporting possible signs of dementia within agreed ways of working

We know that people who may be showing some symptoms of dementia may not recognise or want to acknowledge that there has been a change. Often it is family and friends who begin to notice subtle changes. These may be dismissed at first as 'normal signs of ageing' or mistaken for other problems like depression. Sometimes the carers themselves are in denial and prefer to carry on by masking the problem.

It is important to remain objective when reporting concerns. Do not offer opinions but rather state what is actually happening. For example, do not say 'she is always confused and in a bad mood' rather 'she has forgotten that it is breakfast time over several weeks, she does not remember where her bedroom is and has shouted at staff and residents on each occasion'.

Never use labels or stereotypical language. You must instead use language that is appropriate and person centred. Other professionals may need to read your assessment or care plan so ensure it is:

- **Clear** – do not use jargon or abbreviations.
- **Concise** – keep to the point and do not speculate.

- **Comprehensive** – be thorough, cover the areas that are important for a holistic assessment.
- **Compliant** – make sure you understand and follow your organisation's policies and procedures.

Reporting the first signs of dementia can be done through various channels. The person or the family may go to the GP because they are ready to ask for support. The GP or district nurse may notice signs and symptoms and discuss it with the person. It is common for GPs to become concerned because the person begins to contact the GP surgery on a frequent basis, or alternatively they forget appointments. The GP may raise these concerns with the patient.

If the person is supported at home by domiciliary services, or attends a day centre, signs of dementia may be noted by staff. It is important in all these circumstances to bear in mind that the person's permission must be sought before a referral to the GP can be made.

It is also common for people who are admitted to hospital who show signs of confusion to have a further assessment. Delirium must be ruled out, and if the medical staff are concerned that the symptoms suggest other mental health problems they may consider a referral either to the GP or direct to secondary mental health services for a further assessment.

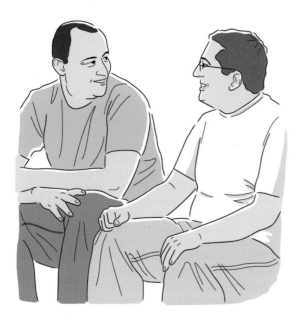

Figure 1.9 Communicating effectively is very important when assessing the person with dementia.

Processes of reporting possible signs of dementia may differ slightly in different areas of the country. Patient confidentiality must be observed and in most cases the consent of the person must be sought before the referral is made.

Evidence activity

 2.3 The process of reporting possible signs of dementia

Think about the professional people you come across in your work. How might these people see the symptoms of dementia and how would they report their concerns?

2.4 Describe the possible impact of receiving a diagnosis of dementia on:

The individual with dementia

The impact of telling someone their diagnosis can be softened by focusing on the strengths and skills of the person. Respect for their positive attributes promotes feelings of:

- **Inclusion** – because of the stigma, some people with dementia feel that they are excluded from their usual networks. It is important to emphasise that they may have dementia, but they also 'have a life' and the right to access services and facilities like anyone else.
- **Empowerment** – a diagnosis of dementia does not make them less of a person. They may need to make some adjustments in their life but strengths and talents must not be underestimated.
- **Participation** – people with dementia can still make a powerful contribution to their family, their wider social network and even to society.

It is important to help the person through the barriers that stigma creates, to reassure them that they can live well with dementia and that by looking after themselves mentally and physically they can continue to live a fulfilling life. Most of all, the person must not feel alone in their dementia. Practical and emotional support is vital in softening the blow.

Family and friends

The shock of the diagnosis is often associated with the stigma attached to dementia. Life changes instantly and plans and dreams can be compromised. The wife or husband, son or daughter may envisage a long road ahead as a carer, unable to live life to the full. In short, it was not what they expected and so they are unprepared. They may need to stop work or juggle other family commitments. This can have an impact financially, emotionally and physically.

> ## Time to reflect
>
> **2.4** The possible impact of receiving a diagnosis of dementia
>
> If you were to receive a diagnosis of dementia, what support information and advice would you want to receive? What emotions might you experience?

LO3 Understand how dementia care must be underpinned by a person centred approach

3.1 Compare a person centred and a non-person centred approach to dementia care

We will look more fully at person centred care in Chapter 2, DEM 202 and DEM 204.

We put the person with dementia at the centre of our work with them. We take a holistic view, ensuring that we assess and plan for their needs by taking into account their preferences, rights as a citizen and their needs. We do not adopt the medical model, seeing dementia as a problem to be solved. Rather we look at the person and support them to overcome or manage the barriers in their way.

To be able to deliver a person centred approach we must:

- Know and understand the process and experience of dementia.
- Fully assess the person, ensuring we have considered their needs, rights and preferences.

- Treat the person with dignity and respect.
- Have looked at issues of positive risk-taking and choice.
- Value their personhood (individuality).
- Ensure their physical needs are met.
- Support them in their emotional, spiritual and social needs.
- Accept them as they are and enter into 'their world' using appropriate communication techniques.
- Provide a socially and intellectually stimulating environment.

A person centred approach does not necessarily take into account what others may think. For example, the person may have managed to dress themselves, but in mismatching clothes. This is not important – what is important is the fact they have done so independently, have a sense of achievement and wellbeing and feel empowered. It would be a negative intervention to try to make the person change their clothes unless their dignity was compromised. Our role is to support the person and a family member who may find it difficult to come to terms with the fact that their mother is happy wearing clothes that do not match, for example. This is not to say that we do not respect the choices the person may have made when they had more capacity. For example a man may always have worn a suit. We should continue to respect that choice unless they indicate otherwise.

A non-person centred approach to dementia care is more task oriented. The person is seen as a series of 'things to do', including personal care, meal times, and bedtimes and so on. The focus is on the staff routine rather than the process of the person's day. In a non-person centred approach the person is expected to comply with routines and systems which probably mean very little to them. They are expected to eat in noisy dining rooms when they have probably always eaten alone. They may be expected to get dressed before breakfast, when in fact it was always their habit to eat first. Such regimes do not use life stories to inform the staff and there is little acknowledgement of the individuality of each person. This approach is documented as having a negative impact on people with dementia. They can become withdrawn or agitated because so little meaningful time is spent with them.

> 'Opportunities for activity and engagement have a huge impact on quality of life and affect important outcomes including mortality, yet over half of carers felt the person they cared for did not have enough to do during the day in the home.'
>
> ('Home from Home', Alzheimer's society 2007)

Research and investigate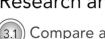

(3.1) Compare a person centred and a non-person centred approach to dementia care

Find out about 'Home from Home' an Alzheimer's society report into the care of people with dementia in care homes. What are the main messages of the report?

(3.2) Describe a range of different techniques that can be used to meet the fluctuating abilities and needs of the individual with dementia

In a person centred approach techniques should be chosen to meet the needs of the individual – what works for one person may not for another. Here are a range of techniques and activities which may be beneficial:

- Improvements and repairs – rewiring, widening doors, specially designed shower facilities.
- Sources of financial and legal advice, and advocacy.
- Information sources, libraries, internet, local voluntary organisations.
- Services arranged by local authorities known as 'community care services' may include: home care services, respite care, signposting services.
- Equipment and adaptations – specialist cutlery, raised toilet seats, wheelchairs, ramps, grab rails, continence equipment, dossett boxes for medication, medic alert bracelets.
- Assistive technology – medication carousels, door sensors, flood detectors, carbon monoxide detectors.
- Memory aids – easy to see clocks, calendars, newspapers, diaries, notice boards and telephone reminders.
- Voluntary organisations provide services such as information, helplines, support groups, lunch clubs and home care schemes.
- Activities and relaxation techniques, including music therapy, aromatherapy, 'singing for the brain', circle dancing, tai chi, reminiscence activities.
- Encouraging 'normal' household activities like folding towels, setting tables, dusting, lacing shoes, making pastry, winding wool, reading the newspaper.
- 'Validation' of meaningful occupation – if the person is actively replicating an activity from their past life this should not be discouraged – it may seem meaningless to you, but in the context of their memory it is important to them. This could be anything from polishing a spoon to tidying paperwork. Think about the person's life story – what did they do as an occupation?

Case Study

(3.2) Mrs Brown

Mrs Brown is admitted to hospital for a minor operation. She has vascular dementia. She used to be a waitress and she likes to keep busy all day. She is quite distressed in the unfamiliar environment.

What techniques and possible activities could you suggest to the ward staff to help her settle?

(3.3) Describe how myths and stereotypes related to dementia may affect the individual and their carers

A myth is a legend or a fairy story and a stereotype is a way of categorising people according to their shared aspects.

Dementia myths include:

- it is a consequence of ageing
- poor memory is part of getting old
- dementia means you are not intelligent
- dementia is caused by eating food cooked in aluminium saucepans
- people with dementia are always violent.

Dementia stereotypes include:

- people are always incontinent
- people are dishevelled
- people cannot work

- people are 'gaga'
- people cannot communicate.

Such myths and legends perpetuate (carry on) the fear of dementia which means that people with dementia and their families are often afraid of telling others about their condition. They can become socially excluded because of the lack of knowledge and understanding from others. The stigma of such a diagnosis can prevent people from seeking advice and support quickly enough. They may avoid social events and have to cope with their social network shrinking as friends and family avoid coming to terms with the condition.

Evidence activity

 Myths and stereotypes related to dementia

Produce a poster for display in a public area that highlights the various myths and stereotypes associated with dementia and describes why they are unfounded.

 Describe ways in which individuals and carers can be supported to overcome their fears

We know that a combination of lack of public and professional awareness, late diagnosis, negative media images, myths, stereotypes and negative experiences all contribute to a general fear of dementia.

Recently, dementia awareness campaigns have recognised this fear, and aim to improve public and professional awareness and understanding of dementia. These campaigns raise awareness that dementia is common and it is not an inevitable consequence of ageing. They also provide information on how to seek help and what treatment is available.

Stigma and fears are addressed by explaining that someone with dementia is no less a person, that dementia is not an immediate death sentence, that life can be lived well with dementia and that people with dementia can continue to make a positive contribution.

Dementia awareness campaigns encourage healthy lifestyles and promote health checks and early diagnosis.

Celebrity status has also been used to promote campaigns.

At more local levels primary care services (GPs), secondary care services (mental health services) and voluntary and independent organisations as well as social services are working together more to support people with dementia and their carers. In response to the National Dementia Strategy, there is a big education campaign underway as well as new willingness to work together to provide more comprehensive support and services.

Evidence activity

Design a leaflet aimed at carers and friends of people with dementia which aims to give a 'user friendly' explanation of dementia and promotes the positive message of living well with dementia.

Time to reflect

What do you think about dementia? Will the way you treat a person with dementia change now that you have read this chapter? What will change and why?

Useful websites

www.dementia2010.org
www.personcentredccareadvocate.org
www.alzheimers.org.uk
www.dementiauk.org
www.direct.gov.uk
www.carers.org

Assessment Summary DEM 301

Reading this unit and completing the activities will have provided you with knowledge, understanding and skills required to improve your awareness of the process and experience of dementia.

To achieve the unit, your assessor will require you to:

Learning Outcomes	Assessment Criteria
1 Understand the neurology of dementia	**1.1** Describe a range of causes of dementia syndrome See evidence activity 1.1, page 15
	1.2 Describe the types of memory impairment commonly experienced by individuals with dementia See evidence activity 1.2, page 16
	1.3 Explain the way that individuals process information with reference to the abilities and limitations of individuals with dementia See case study 1.3, page 17
	1.4 Explain how other factors can cause changes in an individual's condition that may not be attributable to dementia See evidence activity 1.4, page 17
	1.5 Explain why the abilities and needs of an individual with dementia may fluctuate See time to reflect 1.5, page 188
2 Understand the impact of recognition and diagnosis of dementia	**2.1** Describe the impact of early diagnosis and follow up to diagnosis See evidence activity 2.1, page 18
	2.2 Explain the importance of recording possible signs or symptoms of dementia in an individual in line with agreed ways of working See case study 2.2, page 20
	2.3 Explain the process of reporting possible signs of dementia within agreed ways of working See evidence activity 2.3, page 21
	2.4 Describe the possible impact of receiving a diagnosis of dementia on: • The individual • Their family and friends See time to reflect 2.4, page 22

Learning Outcomes	Assessment Criteria
3 Understand how dementia care must be underpinned by a person centred approach	(3.1) Compare a person centred approach and a non person centred approach to dementia care See research and investigate 3.1, page 23
	(3.2) Describe a range of different techniques that can be used to meet the fluctuating abilities and needs of the individual with dementia See case study 3.2, page 23
	(3.3) Describe how myths and stereotypes related to dementia may affect the individual and their carers See evidence activity 3.3, page 24
	(3.4) Describe ways in which individuals and carers can be supported to overcome their fears See evidence activity 3.4, page 24

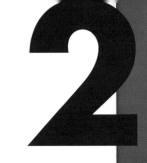

Person Centred Care in Dementia

DEM 202 The person centred approach to the care and support of individuals with dementia

What are you finding out?

This unit will look at the meaning of a person centred approach for people with dementia. We will learn how this approach should run through our everyday work and how to put ideas into practice in **person centred care**. The chapter looks more broadly at relationships in order to understand the place a person with dementia has in their wider social network, and how important this is when we support them.

Some of the activities in this unit are also suitable for DEM 204. Activities will indicate which assessment criteria they are suitable for.

In this unit you will:

• Understand approaches that enable individuals with dementia to experience wellbeing

• Understand the role of carers in the care and support of individuals with dementia

• Understand the roles of others in the support of individuals with dementia

LO1 Understand approaches that enable individuals with dementia to experience wellbeing

Key terms

Wellbeing this means a feeling of self-worth, being able to make decisions for ourselves (self-determination). Having a sense of hope.

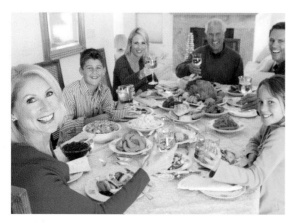

Figure 2.1 Personhood recognises the uniqueness of the individual and the place they have in their family and society.

1.1 Describe what is meant by a person centred approach

A person centred approach to care and support is fundamental to all aspects of health and social care. For people with dementia it is particularly important that we ensure that their individuality, needs, wishes and wellbeing are at the centre of all we do to support them. Put simply, we must always see the person first and then the dementia. No two people are alike so this must be true for someone with dementia. Each person with dementia is an individual with an illness that will affect him or her in different ways. Tom Kitwood talks about the **'personhood'** of people with dementia. He said 'When you have met one

person with dementia you have met one PERSON with dementia' (Tom Kitwood, *Dementia Reconsidered*). This means that although the dementia may affect the way a person thinks and acts, it does not mean that it erodes their individuality or 'personhood'. The way we treat someone with dementia will affect the way they feel and behave. It is important to remember that we must value each individual.

Key terms

Personhood is defined by Tom Kitwood as the recognition, respect and trust given to one individual by others. It is what makes us individuals, unique and with the right of self-determination.

When a person with dementia finds that their mental abilities are declining, they often feel vulnerable and can lack self-esteem. It is important that we offer reassurance and support. The people closest to them – their carers, support staff, friends and family – must help the person with dementia to retain their sense of identity and feelings of self-worth. We must value their sense of reality which may be very different to ours as well as respect their life story and history because these are some of the things which make us unique.

Research and investigate

1.1 (DEM 202) Approaches that enable individuals with dementia to experience wellbeing

Consider those attributes which make us unique as individuals. How do you think we can incorporate them into a person centred approach when working with a person with dementia?

Person centred approaches mean that we cannot view people with dementia in a traditional **stereotypical** way. As a society we can be seen to view older people as 'sweet', or 'cantankerous' or eccentric and so on. This can be seen in the media, for example.

Research and investigate

1.1 (DEM 204)

Describe some examples of stereotypes of older people. What do they tell you about society's view of older people, and in particular older people with dementia?

A person centred approach values older people in a way that reduces **stigma** and sees the individual for who they are, not who we perceive them to be. People with dementia have the same rights as all citizens in society. This includes the right to be treated with dignity and respect.

Key terms

Stigma describes the way in which we look at people in a negative way, for example we might associate dementia with challenging behaviour and make an assumption that everyone who has dementia must be aggressive or verbally abusive. We stigmatise people by associating them with negative aspects of their disability, we make assumptions about people and consequently demonstrate a lack of respect for them, as well as taking away their dignity.

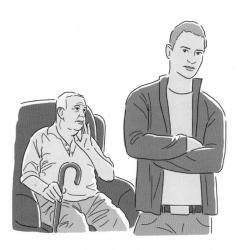

Figure 2.2 Stigma describes the way we make assumptions about people because of their age, skin colour, ethnic origin and so on. It has a negative influence on the way we treat other people.

This is a quote from a person with Alzheimer's disease. It is from **The National Dementia Strategy** and describes the stigma attached to dementia.

> 'It's as though that's it, you are dribbling and nodding, and that's Alzheimer's. That's the picture of Alzheimer's. But we are all sitting here talking perfectly normally. We have got Alzheimer's of some form, we are not nodding and dribbling.'

The National Care Forum describes standards that meet a person centred approach. It explains that this is important to everyone involved, including friends, family, carers and the wider network. This is called a **holistic** approach

Key terms

Holistic is a way of ensuring we look at the whole picture, taking into account all sides of a situation, rather than a one-dimensional view.

This should be an approach to care and support, and not merely a way of writing a care plan. Person centred planning was an approach introduced in the 2001 **'Valuing People'** Strategy for people with learning disabilities. Person centred care tends to be a term more widely used in dementia care. The culture of any service – a care home, or domiciliary service or a team of volunteers, for example, should all have the same values, that is, to put the person with dementia at the centre of any support they offer.

The **personalisation** agenda supports this by promoting a way of thinking about services in a different way. It starts with the person rather than the service. It means that we shape support to suit people's individual needs. Personalisation is about making universal services accessible to all. This means that we should no longer rely on traditional kinds of services and expect a person with dementia to fit into them. For example, not everyone will want to go to a day centre. Instead everyone regardless of their need or disability should have an equal right to use services available to everyone, for example, health clubs, art clubs or the local café.

We make sure that people are given as much information as possible about services and are supported to make informed decisions about their care and support.

We ensure we are supporting people earlier in their illness or disability through early intervention, **re-enablement** and prevention and we recognise and support the role of carers.

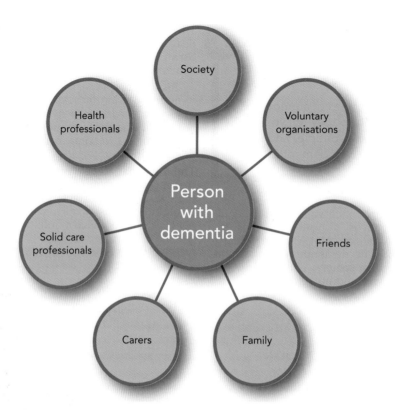

Figure 2.3 A person centred approach ensures that the person with dementia is at the centre of our interaction and takes into account the influence of family and society.

Key terms

Re-enablement means timely episodes of social care support, focusing on skills for daily living, which can enable people to live more independently and reduce their need for ongoing homecare or going into long-term care.

Evidence activity

1.2 (DEM 204) Re-enablement and wellbeing

What do you think are the main problems for someone with dementia in terms of re-enablement? Does re-enablement always fit into their person centred care – and if not, how can we ensure that a person with dementia is receiving the appropriate support?

1.2 Outline the benefits of working with an individual with dementia in a person centred manner

Maintaining a sense of identity

Our sense of who we are is closely connected to the names we call ourselves. It is vital that we address the person with dementia in the way *they* prefer. We should never automatically revert to first names **or** assume that the name you see on a referral form, for example, is their **preferred** name. We must also respect the fact that as short-term memory diminishes the person with dementia might forget your name or use one that is more familiar to them and which they might associate with the way they feel when you interact with them. It is important to respect these feelings and respond positively to this. We must be flexible and show **empathy**.

We also maintain our identity in many other ways, in the way we speak, for example. We might wear particular clothing or jewellery, wear our hair in a particular way, or use body language. (We will talk more about ways of communicating in Chapter 3, DEM 205, DEM 210, DEM 308 and DEM 312.)

Respecting personal values and cultures

It is important that we understand the person's cultural and/or religious background – we need a sense of their personal history and what is important to them. This does not just apply to religious traditions but also to the way they like to be addressed, how they view the world, how they like to dress and so on.

Research and investigate

1.2 (DEM 202) Working with an individual with dementia in a person centred way

Find out about different cultural and religious experiences. Think about how these differences would affect the ways you would interact with people.

Maintaining dignity and privacy

This is key to all our values when working in a person centred way. It is a fundamental human right to be treated with dignity and to have our privacy respected. The Social Care Institute for Excellence (SCIE) describes dignity as follows:

'Dignity consists of many overlapping aspects, involving respect, privacy, autonomy.

Standard dictionary definition: a state, quality or manner worthy of esteem or respect; and ...self-respect. Dignity in (person centred) care, therefore, means the kind of care, in any setting, which supports and promotes, and does not undermine, a person's self-respect regardless of any difference.'

We have already noted that people with dementia can have a weaker sense of self-worth because they realise that they are not as independent as

before, and perhaps not able to contribute to society or their family as they used to. They see their skills and knowledge sets fading as their memory begins to deteriorate and this leads to feelings of frustration, helplessness and anxiety. They may feel worthless and inadequate. It is therefore important to respect and if appropriate acknowledge those feelings and treat the person with dignity and courtesy, whatever the situation. Offer reassurance and support but be careful not to 'talk down' to the person. Person centred care means that we take into account the feelings of the person. They may need you to acknowledge their sadness or frustration and if so it is important to demonstrate that you have empathy.

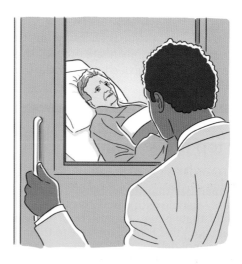

Figure 2.4 It is important that the dignity and privacy of the individual is maintained at all times. Think about how you would feel if you were the person in bed.

correct but rather concentrate on what the person *can* do rather than what they cannot do. Help the person to have positive feelings about themselves by acknowledging achievements and respecting their feelings.

Respecting privacy may be more tricky in a care home and therefore it is very important to be aware of the principles of respecting dignity as a care group.

Research and investigate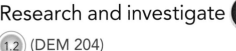

1.2 (DEM 204)

Research the national 'Dignity In Care Campaign' at dignityincare.org.uk. This is a national campaign led by the Department of Health.

Ten top tips for a person centred approach

1. Remember that dementia is an organic illness – people with dementia may behave in a way that other people find difficult to manage – this is probably due to their illness and is not deliberate.
2. Try to understand why they are behaving in a particular way and that they remain a unique person.
3. Dementia affects people in different ways.
4. The person may rely on past rather than recent memories – respect that and communicate in a way that helps them have a sense of wellbeing.
5. Help the person feel valued and respected.
6. Never argue – agree and distract and divert.
7. Never lecture – reassure.
8. Never say I told you so – repeat.
9. Never say you can't – encourage people to do what they can.
10. Never demand or command – model /show and ask.

(Extract from Alzheimers' Society 10 top tips of care giving.)

Evidence activity

These tips could be transferred onto a poster or bookmark or a card to keep in your pocket, as a good way of reminding yourself and others about good person centred care.

What is person centred care?

- It is when we recognise a person's individuality and we respect and value their life story, that is their personal history.
- It is when we understand and empathise with the perspective and experiences of the person with dementia.
- It is when we support the person in maintaining their individuality and independence whenever possible by focusing on what the person can do, not what they can't.

Time to reflect

1.2 (DEM 202 and DEM 204)
Working with an individual with dementia in a person centred way

Think about the service you work in or one that you have some experience of. What evidence is there to show the service is person centred? How can you contribute to improving that person centred approach?

LO2 Understand the role of carers in the care and support of individuals with dementia

Now we will move on to think about those people who support the person with dementia. A carer is not necessarily a family member. Supporting a person with dementia can be very demanding and we will look at both the positive and negative aspects of this role for the carer as well as the 'cared for' person.

2.1 Describe the role that carers have in the care and support of individuals with dementia

Two thirds of people with dementia live at home, and many of them will rely on another person for support in a variety of ways.

We can use the term 'carer' in two specific ways. Carers are sometime referred to as 'care givers' and relate to those people who are family members, partners, friends and neighbours who give support and care to a person with dementia but who are usually unpaid. They are not necessarily women. The traditional role of carer fell to the woman but as we change as a society, so the role of carers is changing.

It should also be noted that some families do not see themselves as 'carers' with separate roles, but rather view it as a natural or 'integral' part of family life. We must therefore always be sensitive to the culture of families and to the existing relationships within the family.

Carers are part of the wider network of holistic care and it is important that as paid 'professional' carers we both understand and respect their role. It is important that we work together in partnership rather than always thinking 'we know best'. It is also true that some people are 'expert carers' and we must always respect the views and feelings of carers and take this into account when building up a picture of the situation of the person with dementia and their care giver.

However, it is not always the case that carers initially adopt their role with a wide knowledge of dementia, and it is part of our role to support and signpost them to information and advice. We should make sure that anyone involved in caring for the person with dementia has as much relevant information as possible. This will help in person centred approaches to care and support.

Issues faced by carers

It would be misleading to think that all carers are either happy or comfortable in their caring role, or that they always have the best interests of the cared for person at the centre of what they do. It would also be true to say that some carers feel anger, or sadness or guilt. When we are in a professional role it is part of our responsibility not only to support carers when they need it, but also to recognise problems experienced by carers. The impact that dementia has on the relationship between the person and the family member is crucial. There may be a sense of loss or confusion over the behaviour of the person with dementia. The carer may also be placed in a situation where they have to carry out the role of decision maker. It is only really in the last 15 to 20 years that family carers and their needs have been acknowledged as a social care issue.

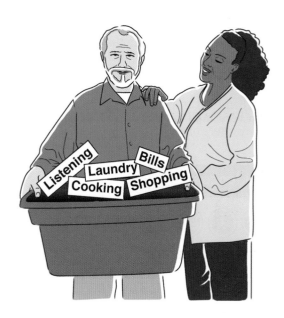

Figure 2.5 Carers have to face many issues every day and their caring role can be a matter of juggling priorities. It is important that we offer support.

The Association of Directors of Adult Social Services (ADASS) produced a 'good practice' paper in which they say that some practitioners (professional carers) work to a 'rule of optimism'. This means that we can overestimate families and friends' ability or wish to care, and this can sometimes lead to forms of neglect, which if not supported adequately could lead to a form of abuse.

Here are two examples of possible abuse:

1. When the person with dementia has care needs that the carer cannot cope with.

   Example: This might include situations where personal care needs like incontinence or eating are so great that the carer is unsure how to manage without help, but are afraid to ask for that support. Their greatest fear is that if they are seen to be 'failing' because then they will be persuaded that the solution is to move their family member into a care home. They are not deliberately neglecting the person with dementia, but as a carer they need a lot of support. Without that support the situation will probably deteriorate.

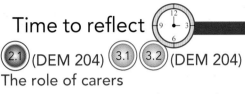

Time to reflect

 (DEM 204)   (DEM 204)

The role of carers

Think about a situation where you have supported a carer. What were the issues for them? Were there other people who could support them – what was their role?

2. When the carer manages all aspects of care to very high standards and will not accept any offers of help from services.

Evidence activity

 (DEM 204)

The role of carers

Describe the issues that could arise from this situation described in point 2 for:

- the person with dementia
- the carer.

Discuss this scenario with a social worker or your manager. In what ways could you support this carer?

There can be many aspects to the role of a carer, including the following.

Practical support

This type of support includes those tasks associated with 'activities of daily living' (ADLs). People with dementia may begin to experience difficulty using money, or finding their way, or making their wishes known. **Shopping** can become a problem and it is often one of the first things a carer may help with because it is soon very noticeable when a person is not shopping or eating well. However, we must remember that the person has the right to **choice** and self-determination so it is vital that they are involved in the decisions about what food to buy and so on.

Dementia causes problems with short-term memory loss and sequencing (doing things in the right order). **Housework** can therefore be a problem. Again, this soon becomes noticeable to the family member, friend or neighbour. People with dementia may simply forget to clean their

home, or may do the same task repeatedly. There are issues for both the person with dementia and the carer though. Keeping your house clean and tidy can be a very sensitive issue. We all have different standards, and we should never impose our own standards on other people. A person with dementia, for example, may always have been untidy. A carer may be tempted to 'sort things out' but this might not be the right approach. Remember: this is the person's own home and we must respect their **privacy**. It is important not to take over but rather to work with the person with dementia.

Managing finances can also be problematic. Bills might be forgotten and go unpaid, the person may find difficulty in managing large amounts of money or understanding how to pay at a shop. Carers often help in these situations and may need to make arrangements with the bank or other agencies to protect themselves and the person with dementia. The most common way to allow carers to access the person's money is through direct debits or standing orders. Many banks and building societies now offer an easy-to-use basic bank account. Pensions or benefits can be paid directly into these accounts. With most basic bank accounts you can set up direct debits (e.g. to pay regular bills) and standing orders (e.g. to make a regular payment of the same amount to someone).

Financial abuse is one of the most common types of abuse and therefore all those involved need protection. It might require an application for '**Lasting Power of Attorney**'.

Research and investigate

 (DEM 202) (DEM 204)

Care and support of individuals with dementia

Find out about the Lasting Powers of Attorney and how this can help both the person with dementia as well as support the carer in helping the person to manage their finances. **Age UK factsheet 22 October 2010** is a very useful reference.

People with dementia may have difficulty remembering **appointments with their GP, hospital, bank and so on**. They may also have problems **using public transport**. Carers often take responsibility for ensuring these appointments are kept, and for transporting the person. Details discussed at the appointment are easily forgotten for someone with short-term memory loss and their carer might take responsibility for managing these situations. It can be all too easy to 'take over' and again the **rights** of the person with dementia must be respected. They must also be encouraged to have some control over their plans and to use memory joggers – notebooks and diaries, for example.

Another problem encountered by people with dementia is **managing meal preparation**. They may forget when to eat, or how to cook a meal. Neighbours and family will often take on this task. There are other organisations who can help. There may be a local 'meals on wheels' service or companies who will deliver microwaveable meals. These services can prevent over-reliance on the carer as well as giving the person with dementia some control and choice.

People with dementia may begin to need help first with these practical domestic tasks, rather than personal care, for example. They can continue to enjoy many activities though, and carers should be supported in helping the person benefit from these, rather than assuming they are unable to do anything. Such tasks might include everyday things like cleaning shoes, drying the dishes or folding laundry. It is our role as professional carers to educate family members, neighbours and friends to support the person in ways that will empower them and raise their self-esteem. Good person centred care planning will help to involve everyone in this.

Support with personal care

This is probably one of the most sensitive aspects of supporting someone with dementia. It can be a very daunting and distressing idea for the son or daughter of someone with dementia. It feels as if roles are reversed, and that being the case, the dignity of the person with dementia is crucial. This may be one area where the carer needs most support from us and it is important that we base this on a detailed assessment and understanding of the needs of the person with dementia.

They may neglect their personal hygiene – they may forget to wash, or struggle to sequence tasks – putting clothes on in the wrong order or forgetting the process of brushing teeth. Incontinence of urine and/or faeces may be an issue and although the person with dementia might be unaware of the problem, their carer could be embarrassed or angry about the situation. We therefore have to help with the task in a person centred way, but we also need to deal with the feelings of the carer who may not understand why this is happening to their friend or family member.

A carer who helps someone with dementia in all these aspects of daily life can become very tired and frustrated. They may experience guilt that they cannot do more, or anxiety that things seem out of their control. Added to all this they will probably be offering **emotional support**.

Some of the main symptoms of dementia include:

- loss of memory
- communication problems
- mood changes
- loss of functioning
- becoming reliant on other people.

These symptoms can all lead the person with dementia to experience a variety of feelings. These might include sadness, loneliness, frustration, anger and depression. As well as dealing with their own emotions, the carer also has to offer support, patience and acceptance to the person with dementia. It is vital that the carer listens to the person with dementia. These emotions should be acknowledged.

We expect the carer to show empathy and to accept 'odd' behaviour. We expect them to exercise patience and understand how the person with dementia is feeling. In the later stages of the illness they may be in a position where they have to listen to the same conversation constantly or where they have to change soiled sheets several times in the night, or reassure someone that they are safe. All this can take its toll. So how can we support the carer?

2.2 Explain the value of developing a professional working relationship with carers

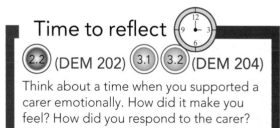

Time to reflect

2.2 (DEM 202) 3.1 3.2 (DEM 204)

Think about a time when you supported a carer emotionally. How did it make you feel? How did you respond to the carer?

Think about your attitude and behaviour. What might you now change in your practice? A practical way of supporting carers is by finding out about their specific issues and needs. Completing a carer's assessment can do this.

This is an example of the questions a carer might be asked by a support worker (this could be a social worker or a nurse, for example) in order to establish what the needs of the carer are. Under the **Carers' Recognition Act** it is the responsibility of the Local Authority to offer carer assessments

Carers' Assessment

If you are a "carer"- if you look after a relative or friend who needs support to live at home, your local Social Services may be able to help make things easier for you or put you in touch with an organisation that can help. We may be able to provide services to the person you care for or for you.

We need to have a discussion with you to work out which services would best meet your need. We need to think about:

What help does the person you care for need?

What help are you giving them at the moment?

To do this it is a good idea to think about the following questions:

Do you get enough sleep?

Is your health affected in other ways?

Are you able to get out and about?

Do you get any time for yourself?

Are your other relationships affected?

Do you want information about benefits?

Are you worried you may have to give up?

Services that might help you

Services that give you a break

Emotional support from other carers or people who understand

Help with household tasks

Help with caring tasks during the day/night

Things to consider:

Your understanding of your family member's needs – would you like more information and advice?

Other pressures on your family, work and other commitments – are you able to go to work as usual, or shop or enjoy a social life? Are you able to spend time with your family?

Information or advice about returning to work or retraining issues

Financial problems – does being in a caring role restrict you from going to work? Do you have additional expenses because of caring for someone?

Need for practical help

Contingency Planning – for example have you been able to make plans in case of emergency?

Figure 2.6 Carers are entitled to a carer's assessment to help them identify their needs and issues.

Case Study

     (DEM 202)

 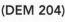 **(DEM 204)**

Ruby

Ruby lives in a small terraced house in a small market town. She has been diagnosed with Alzheimer's disease, after she visited the Memory Service with her husband, Charlie. Their son and daughter live in the next town, 10 miles away.

Charlie and Ruby have never relied on other people and Charlie is worried that now people will want to take over. Ruby is becoming more forgetful and irritable. Charlie is finding it increasingly difficult to persuade her to wash and change her clothes. Their daughter, Mandy, visits once a week and is cross with her father for not doing more for mum, but Charlie insists that he can only do as much as Ruby will let him. Mandy also notices that her mum and dad are losing weight and suspects that they are living off

snacks. She also thinks that mum is finding it more difficult to get upstairs and noticing bedding in the lounge, asks her dad if this is the case. Charlie is very upset and says that he cannot cope but that Mandy is interfering and he just wants to stay at home with Ruby.

Think about the case study and answer the following questions. It may be helpful to use the carer's assessment as a prompt. You might also find it helpful to discuss with colleagues.

- What are the different issues for Ruby, the person with dementia?
- Charlie, Ruby's main carer – what emotions and difficulties is he experiencing?
- What about Mandy, who is concerned about both her parents?
- What organisations might be able to help?
- Can you think of some professions who could support the family?
- What kind of support would you as a professional offer to Mandy and why?

LO3 Understand the roles of others in the care and support of individuals with dementia

In this section we will learn how the role of health and social care staff can support the person with dementia and their carer. Voluntary organisations like the Alzheimer's Society also have a vital role to play, and often offer information, support and social activities.

  Describe the roles of others and explain when it may be necessary to refer to others when supporting individuals with dementia

3.3 **Explain how to access the additional support of others when supporting individuals with dementia**

Research and investigate

3.1 **3.2** The role of carers

Research the legislation (law) that has been passed to support carers. This includes the Carers (Recognition Services) Act 1995.

Health services

Most mental health services are provided by the NHS and are called 'secondary care services'. Usually they are accessed through the local GP, who will make a referral for the patient. Services vary in different parts of the country, although most areas will have inpatient mental health facilities and community services. These can include Community Mental Health Teams (CMHTs), Memory Services, Day Services and more specialist outreach teams. For example, some areas have 'Rapid Response' or 'Intensive Home Treatment' teams to support people who need urgent support in the community, or Care Home Liaison Teams who specifically help care homes in the care of people with dementia. People with dementia might be supported by a combination of health practitioners. Some will have specialist mental health knowledge.

Mental Health Nurse

The Mental Health Nurse (Registered Mental Nurse, RMN) will usually work in an inpatient unit (ward) or a Community Mental Health Team. The RMN working in the community supports older people with a wide range of mental health problems, including dementia. They visit people in their own homes and their primary role is to:

1. Assess the person's mental health needs, taking into account the needs of the carer.

2. Support the person with an appropriate care plan, including liaising with other agencies like social services.

3. Help in the treatment of the person with dementia, by monitoring the effects of medication and other interventions, supporting and educating the carer as well as dealing with changes and new difficulties.

It may be necessary to involve the Mental Health Nurse when the needs of the person with dementia are becoming more complex and there are associated behavioural difficulties. They work closely with families.

Psychiatrist

The psychiatrist is a medically qualified doctor who diagnoses mental illness and prescribes and recommends treatment for the patient. They discuss treatment plans with other practitioners, the patient and their families. Psychiatrists work both on the wards and in the community. They also have specific duties under the Mental Health Act. Most referrals to psychiatrists are made by GPs.

Psychologist

The psychologist is also a medically qualified doctor who deals particularly in cognition, which is the act of knowing. They assess how well a person with dementia is able to use thought processes, memory, problem solving and the use of language. They also look at behavioural issues.

Speech and language therapist (SALT)

The role of a speech and language therapist is to assess and treat people with speech, language and communication problems to enable them to communicate more effectively. They can also work with people who have eating and swallowing problems. These issues affect people with dementia and it is important to refer to the speech and language therapist if the person is having difficulty chewing and swallowing food. The SALT will be able to carry out a swallowing assessment and advise on the safest ways to support the person with their diet. As part of their role speech and language therapists are trained to support people with dementia.

Occupational therapist (OT)

Occupational therapists enable people to perform meaningful and purposeful activities. They work with people with dementia to help them maintain activities of daily living. They can help with improving or maintaining motor functions (the act of performing a task). Their goal is to maintain the person's independence as much as possible. The OT often is asked to advise on someone's safety in their own home. They can help with strategies to minimise risk and to make adjustments to the home to enable the person with dementia to remain at home for as long as possible. Some OTs work in specialist mental health teams.

Physiotherapist

Physiotherapists help and treat people with physical problems. They are healthcare professionals who help people with movement such as walking, sitting and standing. People with dementia may also experience physical problems as well as have symptoms of depression and anxiety. The physiotherapist can help by supporting someone to exercise, or use relaxation techniques. Like OTs, some physiotherapists work in specialist mental health teams.

General Practitioner (GP)

The GP is often the first medical person to be contacted when there is concern that a person is showing signs of cognitive impairment or dementia. The GP works in **Primary Care** Services. The National Dementia Strategy sets out goals for the early diagnosis of dementia and GPs have a critical role to play in this. Mental health services work closely with GPs in the care of someone with dementia. GPs will often support mental health services in monitoring the effects of medication (see Chapter 7) as well as monitoring the progress of someone's dementia.

GPs also have an important role in supporting carers. They may be the first person a carer will turn to and the GP will consider both the issues for the carer and the person with dementia. GPs often 'signpost' patients, that is they will either refer them for support to organisations like social care (social services, adult services) or give them information about other sources of help.

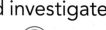

Key terms

Primary Care The Department of Health defines Primary Care as 'services provided by GP practices, dental practices, community pharmacies and high street optometrists'.

Social services or adult services

Like the services provided by the NHS these are called 'statutory services'. This means they are services provided by the state rather than a private (independent) or voluntary organisation. Social services assess people who have social care needs. These could include accommodation, personal care needs, financial difficulties, suspected abuse, carer issues, and assessing for the use of equipment or technology to support someone's independence. They will also look at the best way of working with other organisations. Social services do provide some services like domiciliary care or care homes and extra care housing, but they also work with the private and voluntary sector who provide support to people in their own homes or run care homes.

Social workers are usually employed by social services. Some mental health teams also have social workers in them. Specialist mental health social workers might also have responsibilities under the Mental Health Act. They are called 'Approved Mental Health Professionals' (AMHP). Other qualified staff can also be an AMHP. This means that they assess a person who may need to be detained under the Mental Health Act. Social workers may also work as 'best interest assessors'. They will independently assess a person who may lack capacity, to ensure that the decisions made with or for them are in their 'best interest'.

Research and investigate

(2.3) (DEM 204) The role of others in care and support

Find out about The Mental Capacity Act 2005 and best interests at www.best interests.org.uk.

Social workers will carry out needs assessments for the person with dementia and their carer. They will work with them to look at the best way of meeting those needs. As part of the personalisation agenda they will take a person centred approach. People who have had their needs assessed can then be offered a personal budget to use as they wish to meet their needs. This means they are given more choice and control.

Social workers also work closely with other professionals and often carry out joint assessments. They also signpost people to other services.

Voluntary organisations

These are usually charitable organisations. This means they are 'not for profit'. They might employ both paid staff and volunteers. In most areas of the country some voluntary organisations are 'commissioned' to provide services. This means that the local health trust agrees to fund them to deliver particular services. These might include lunch clubs, befriending services or a care navigator role. Voluntary organisations often complement the role of statutory services.

The Alzheimer's Society is a national charity which campaigns for people with dementia, provides direct services and also provides education programmes. They also support carers. Mental health professionals and social workers often refer people with dementia and their families to the Alzheimer's Society so that they can access additional support and advice. You can find their website address at the end of the chapter.

Research and investigate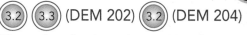

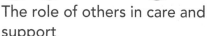 (3.2) (3.3) (DEM 202) (3.2) (DEM 204)

The role of others in care and support

Find your local branch of the Alzheimer's Society. What services do they provide for people with dementia? Admiral Nurses, Dementia Care Advisors, and Independent Mental Capacity Advocates are all roles specifically created to help people with dementia. Look on their website to find out more.

Case Study

   (DEM 202)

  (DEM 204)

Mrs Jones

Mrs Jones has developed vascular dementia. She also has a heart condition, which makes her breathless. She forgets that she is not able to get about very well and is often frustrated and angry when her son tries to help her with everyday tasks. She lives in a ground floor flat but her son feels she is struggling to cope. More recently she has been forgetting to eat and take her medication properly and often tells her son to leave when he tries to help. The house is very chaotic, Mrs Jones is unkempt and losing weight, and her mental health is deteriorating. Her son often finds her crying when he visits. She is very suspicious of other people and has refused all offers of help in the past. Currently she sees the psychiatrist every 6 months for a routine check-up. Her next appointment is in three months. Her friend, Ann visits once a week.

These are the views of Mrs Jones, her son and Ann:

Mrs Jones: 'I am frightened because everyone tells me I forget things and should not be here. This is my home and I don't want to go anywhere. I manage OK – they think I am mad. Well, I'm not.'

Son: 'I know she wants to stay here but she can't cope and she doesn't see that because of her dementia. I don't want her to go into care but this can't go on. I am worried to death. She gets so angry.'

Ann: 'She has changed so much it makes me sad. I want the best for her. She might listen to me more if only they would include me in things.'

Demonstrate what you have learnt about person centred care by explaining:

- What are the issues for Mrs Jones, her son and Ann?
- Which organisations or professionals may need to be involved?
- The type of support to be explored, including assessments.
- What are the issues for the agencies that might support her?
- The possible outcomes for Mrs Jones.

Assessment Summary DEM 202

Reading this unit and completing the activities will have provided you with knowledge, understanding and skills required to understand the person centred approach to the care and support of individuals with dementia.

To achieve the unit, your assessor will require you to:

Learning Outcomes	Assessment Criteria
1 Understand approaches that enable individuals with dementia to experience wellbeing	(1.1) Describe what is meant by a person centred approach See research and investigate activity 1.1, page 28
	(1.2) Outline the benefits of working with an individual with dementia in a person centred manner See evidence activity 1.2, page 31
2 Understand the role of carers in the care and support of individuals with dementia	(2.1) Describe the role that carers can have in the care and support of individuals with dementia See evidence activity 2.1, page 34
	(2.2) Explain the value of developing a professional working relationship with carers See evidence activity 2.2, page 34
3 Understand the role of others in the support of individuals with dementia	(3.1) Describe the roles of others in the care and support of individuals with dementia See evidence activity 3.1, page 34
	(3.2) Explain when it may be necessary to refer to others when supporting individuals with dementia See evidence activity 3.2, page 34
	(3.3) Explain how to access the additional support of others when supporting individuals with dementia See research and investigate activity 3.3, page 39

DEM 204 Understand and implement a person centred approach to the care and support of individuals with dementia

What are you finding out?

We will look at the ways in which the person with dementia can be more involved in the decisions about their own care and support. This includes the use of life stories and communication skills. We will also understand the process of managing risk within the care plan and how we involve the carer and others in this planning.

By the end of this unit you will be able to

• Understand the importance of a person centred approach to dementia care and support

• Involve the individual with dementia in planning and implementing their care and support using a person centred approach

• Involve carers and others in the care and support of individuals with dementia

LO1 Understand the importance of a person centred approach to dementia care and support

1.1 Describe what is meant by a person centred approach

Support services should be built on the person's individual strengths and abilities, needs and preferences. They should enable people to retain as much independence as possible while supporting them to feel valued and safe. Therefore this should also include robust risk assessments because a person centred approach will involve **positive risk taking**. Rights and choices must be respected, and as care workers we must enter into a partnership with the person with dementia. There must not be an assumption that the person is unable to make informed choices or be involved in decision-making. Depending on the level of a person's dementia different approaches may have to be taken.

A person centred approach means creating a positive environment to help good care practice. It must involve family and friends and identify skills by concentrating on what the person can do rather than what they can't and therefore making goals in care plans achievable.

Person centred care has been expanded to include **relationship centred care**. This describes a way of seeing the person not only at the centre of our assessment and care planning, but also takes into account the bigger picture, by acknowledging that they are part of different relationships.

Time to reflect

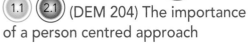 (DEM 204) The importance of a person centred approach

Think about yourself. Make a list of the different types of relationships in your life. Think about someone you have supported. What kinds of relationships do they have? How might this impact on the care and support you provide?

A person and relationship centred approach does not rely on the **medical model of disability**.

A person and relationship centred approach is based more on the social model of disability.

This explains that although people may have a disability (in this case dementia) we do not as a society have to define them like this. The social model says that all people have equal rights – to be heard, to be included, to be consulted and to have access to services.

1.2 Describe how a person centred approach enables individuals with dementia to be involved in their own care and support

If we do not use a person centred approach we are likely to forget that the care and support we give the person with dementia should be based on their life history or story, their likes and dislikes and individual needs. There is a difference between 'perceived' needs and actual needs.

Perceived needs describe the needs of the person that we **assume** they have, looking at the person from our own perspective. We might, for example, assume that the person who is afraid of the dark wants a night light when in fact, if you asked them they would tell you they prefer to leave the curtains open. We may assume that the person who has dementia needs help with dressing when in fact they are perfectly capable so long as we support them to lay their clothes out in the correct order.

A person centred approach means that we communicate with the person in a manner they can respond to and we involve their friends and family in finding out as much as possible about them. By using effective communication skills, life story approaches and a great deal of empathy we can adjust our approach and think about what the person actually needs and what they are telling us.

We can involve the person with dementia in their own care and support by offering choices, respecting their dignity and respecting their individuality. We begin by putting the person at the centre of the assessment and then building a picture of their personal needs and strengths. In the past there has been a tendency to fit services around the person – to assess their needs in terms of the types of support we might have available. For example, we would say that the person needed to go to a day centre rather than thinking about how we meet their expressed need to socialise.

We have talked more about this when describing 'personalisation', which is a way in which we tailor support to fit the person's expressed needs, wishes and strengths.

LO2 Be able to involve the individual with dementia in planning and implementing their care and support using a person centred approach

 Explain how information about personality and life history can be used to support an individual to live well with dementia

Evidence activity

(DEM 204) Information about a person's personality and life history

Talk to a close friend or colleague. Tell them one fact about yourself that they will not know. What is their reaction? They may be surprised or impressed. They may now have a slightly different view of you. Perhaps you have told them you are afraid of something or that you once did a brave act. That new piece of information has added to the jigsaw picture of you and your friend or colleague can use it to help them have a clearer understanding of you.

We can see that generally speaking, the more we know about anyone (not only a person with dementia) the more we understand them and can, if necessary, support them.

There are a variety of ways in which we can learn more and get to know the person with dementia and there are many sources, including:

- the person
- families
- friends and neighbours
- old work colleagues
- other professionals

These people are all part of the person's social network and will, depending on their role, probably see the person in a slightly different way.

Time to reflect

(DEM 204) Information about a person's personality and life history

Think about the 'Mrs Jones' case study on page 40. What are the differences between her son's opinion of her and that of her friend, Ann? What do you think a social worker's view might be? Our own opinions and concerns can influence or colour how we perceive a person with dementia. That is why it is so important to paint a holistic picture and to find out as much as possible from the person at the centre of the care plan – the person with dementia.

Other ways of finding out about the person include 'patient stories'. These are anecdotal accounts of someone's personal experience of their illness and the support they received. In it they might describe how they felt about their care and the people who support them. Patient stories can be used in 'reflective practice', that is a way of understanding and learning from our working practices. Whether we are being truly person centred is a question we should ask ourselves. The way we perceive the support we give and the way it feels for the person on the receiving end can be very different!

The more we understand the person with dementia, the more we can help.

Life history or 'life story' is very popular as a way of getting to know the person with dementia. It has several benefits. Life story work is organic. This means it can grow and change as you gather more information and consequently more insight into the person with dementia. It is therefore not only about 'reminiscing' about the past but is also a way of finding out about the person's likes and dislikes, their fears and hopes and aspirations for the future. You can share a life story in different ways, not just in a scrapbook. A life story resource belongs to that person, not to you or the care home or the service. It does not serve its purpose if it is kept in an office. It should be a well-used possession.

Research and investigate

2.1 (DEM 204) How life stories can help

Find out about the different ways of sharing life stories with people. Describe some of its benefits for people with dementia.

Remember, when helping someone in their life story facts may not seem so important. Memories can be about feelings, so a person may remember how they felt when they first went to the seaside, but might not remember the actual place.

Ideas to talk about include:

- likes and dislikes
- parents
- school
- holidays
- pets
- what makes you laugh/feel sad/cross?
- what have you done that makes you proud?

Time to reflect

2.1 2.2 (DEM 204) Life story work

In your workplace how could you introduce life story work, or improve it if you have started to use it? Who could help you with this?

Remember: not everyone will want to talk about all of these things and there may be some aspects of their life that the person does not want to share. You must respect this and work with the person on the memories and feelings that they feel comfortable with. This is person centred care.

For more information you can go to the website **www.lifestorynetwork.org.uk**.

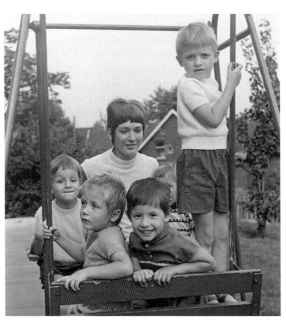

Figure 2.7 People's memories can help define who they are and help us relate to them.

2.2 Communicate with an individual with dementia using a range of methods that meet individuals' abilities and needs

We discuss the different ways of communicating in Chapter 3. If we remember that communication takes several forms, not just verbal language but sounds, body language, music, pictures and so on we can then think about how we apply this to supporting someone in planning and implementing their care. Although we may be required to write a care plan to ensure that we are all aware of the required outcomes for the person with dementia, we can also think more imaginatively about how we express that for the person themselves.

Remember some of the rules of communication:

- Look for clues in the person's behaviour.
- Have good eye contact.
- Mirror body language – respond to the person's emotions.
- Follow up comments rather than asking questions all the time.
- When asking a question, give an option – so 'Do you like roses?' rather than 'what flowers do you like?'.

People may respond to a variety of media. Stimulate the senses by using smells and sound. Music is very evocative of memories and pictures and symbols can be helpful. 'Talking mats' are an example of this. The person may not be able to explain a preference to you but they may be able to point to the relevant picture.

When planning care with a person with dementia, always take into account their previously held views and preferences. They may no longer be able to explain to you how they like to drink their tea or where they prefer to live, but both these things, whether seemingly trivial or major, are important for that person. A personal profile should be used in addition to a care plan. This can give more detail about the person. Think back to Mrs Jones. As her dementia advances her son and friend can help by ensuring that all that relevant information is passed on. Personal profiles can be used in different settings. They are invaluable in care homes but are also a very good way of transferring important information when a person with dementia transfers from one place to another – an admission to hospital, for example.

The Alzheimer's Society produce a profile specifically for this purpose called 'This is me'.

Research and investigate

2.1 (DEM 204) Communicating preferences

Find out if there is similar documentation used in your local hospital or your care setting. If not perhaps you could talk to your manager about implementing something similar.

Some areas that should be covered by a personal profile include

- likes and dislikes
- favourite pasttimes
- personal care needs
- things that make the person anxious.

Evidence activity

2.2 (DEM 204)

How do you think you could 'translate' these ideas into a more person centred approach. For example – 'I am afraid of the dark' or 'I tend to get lost if I am looking for my daughter'.

2.3 2.4 Involving the individual with dementia in identifying and managing risks for their support plan and in opportunities that meet their agreed abilities, needs and preferences

We must use the evidence from several sources. The idea of risk can be very subjective. This means that people see risks very differently. Mrs Jones does not feel she is at risk but her son does because he has more insight. However, we must weigh up the risk because although it may seem risky to us, eliminating the risk may be of no benefit to the person and can disable them further. So we must always be person centred and consider what is in the best interests of the person with dementia.

LO3 Be able to involve carers and others in the care and support of individuals with dementia

Case Study

  (DEM 204) Stella

Stella lives on her own in an old terraced house. She has Alzheimer's disease. She lives in one room most of the time, occasionally pottering into the kitchen to get a drink or a snack. She manages to get upstairs despite her arthritis. Her house is disordered and cramped.

An Occupational Therapist from the local Community Mental Health Team visits her to assess the risks. The GP had visited Stella and was very concerned about her situation.

The OT talked to Stella at length and asked her to show her how she managed.

At the end of the assessment the OT decided to do nothing.

Why do you think the OT made this decision?

Issues to consider when thinking about this scenario:

- Stella had lived in the house all her life.
- She had been going upstairs for many years without falling and was able to show the OT how she got upstairs. She also showed her how she steered her way around her cluttered lounge.
- Although she had a lot of old electrical equipment in the lounge (fires etc.), none of it worked. Stella had a new central heating system.
- There was fresh food in the fridge and evidence from the neighbour that she shopped regularly for Stella.
- The kettle was still warm.

Use your knowledge and understanding to think about the outcome for Stella. The OT acted in a person centred way.

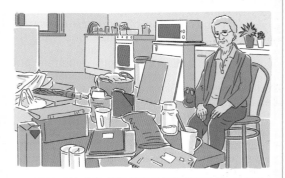

Figure 2.8 We should never make assumptions about how a person lives. It is important to get to know them and make a thorough assessment.

Explain how to increase a carer's understanding of dementia and a person centred approach, and demonstrate how to involve them in the support of a person with dementia

We have already discussed the significant role a carer and others have to play in the support of a person with dementia. We have learnt that we must see them as partners in care and support by acknowledging the advice and knowledge they have about the person. We must also recognise that carers have rights and issues of their own. Traditionally, carers were often seen as working at the edge of care planning – their views may have been taken into account, but there was still a paternalistic view that the 'professional' carers 'knew best'. The move towards person and relationship centred care as well as the personalisation agenda has not only put the person with dementia at the centre it has also acknowledged that carers must be treated as true partners. Indeed, it is often the carer who knows the person with dementia best, and who can give us that vital information that helps us understand the person better.

We can encourage the carer in their understanding of dementia as well as involve them in the support by care planning and consultation.

The Department of Health defines a care plan as:

'essentially about addressing an individual's full range of needs, taking into account their health, personal, social, economic, educational, mental health, ethnic and cultural background and circumstances. It recognises that there are other issues in addition to medical needs that can impact on a person's total health and wellbeing.'

A care plan should be based on an assessment of the person's needs and preferences. All care plans should be outcomes based and needs led.

A care plan should be written so that it will explain how certain results can be achieved. The person may **need** support with shopping but the **outcome** would be to ensure the person continues to eat well, respecting their personal choice of food.

Traditionally, a care plan was written in a way that described the need of the person and therefore it did not really emphasise the positive aspects of someone's life. 'Needs help with personal care, cleaning' suggests a task oriented approach which describes the person almost as a series of jobs to be done and problems to be solved. The introduction of the **personalisation** approach encourages us to look at the individuality of the person, and with the involvement of the person with dementia and their carer we can achieve outcomes that **they** want rather than those we perceive them to need. Hence they can have a more active involvement in their own care plan.

Personalisation means thinking about care and support services in an entirely different way from the task oriented approach and making sure the person with dementia is put first. There has been a tendency to try to 'fit' people into services, rather than to tailor services to meet someone's actual need. For example, we might assume that because a person would like to socialise more they should go to a day centre. This might not be the case. They may prefer to go out to a café to meet a friend or join an exercise class. This is what personalisation is about – giving people more choice and control and the ability to access facilities regardless of their disability. This also takes into account the role the carer has in the plan.

A care plan should be detailed enough for it to be meaningful to the person with dementia and their carer. It should be written in a way that reflects an understanding of the perspective and experiences of the person with dementia. By including the person as much as possible, the process will be more helpful and they are more likely to 'own' the care plan. They may be able to write their own plan with you. Language should be in 'plain English' and technical terms and abbreviations avoided. A care plan should also be responsive – a document where day-to-day outcomes and preferences for care and support are recorded. We need to provide an individualised care plan that is in tune with peoples' changing needs.

In a care plan you may be aiming to achieve such outcomes as:

- the person with dementia being enabled to maintain the relationships with significant others as they choose
- developing a positive relationship and gaining trust and confidence
- encouraging social inclusion
- promoting self-care when possible, including independence and control over support and care.

A care plan might include the following areas:

- personal care needs
- activities of daily living
- relationship issues
- risk and management of risk
- physical health needs
- housing issues
- leisure/ meaningful occupation
- medication needs.

Useful websites

www.dementiauk.org

www.carersuk.org

www.direct.gov.uk

www.nhs.uk/carers

www.alzheimers.org.uk

www.lifestorynetwork.org.uk

www.dh.gov.uk/en/SocialCare/ Deliveringsocialcare/MentalCapacity/IMCA/ index.htm

---

Evidence activity

 (DEM 204) Involving the person with dementia and their carer

Look at the care plans that you currently use. How could you improve them? Think about ways in which you could involve the person with dementia and their carer in a more person and relationship centred way.

Assessment Summary DEM 204

Reading this unit and completing the activities will have provided you with knowledge, understanding and skills required to understand and implement the person centred approach to the care and support of individuals with dementia.

To achieve the unit, your assessor will require you to:

Learning Outcomes	Assessment Criteria
1 Understand the importance of a person centred approach to dementia care and support	**1.1** Describe what is meant by a person centred approach See research and investigate activity 1.1, page 29
	1.2 Describe how a person centred approach enables individuals with dementia to be involved in their own care and support See evidence activities 1.2, pages 30 and 31
2 Be able to involve the individual with dementia in planning and implementing their care and support using a person centred approach	**2.1** Explain how information about personality and life history can be used to support an individual to live well with dementia See evidence activity 2.1, page 43
	2.2 Communicate with an individual with dementia using a range of methods that meet individual needs and abilities See evidence activity 2.2, page 46
	2.3 Communicate with an individual with dementia in identifying and managing risks for their care and support plan See case study 2.3, page 46
	2.4 Involve an individual with dementia in opportunities that meet their agreed abilities, needs and preferences See case study 2.4, page 46
3 Be able to involve carers and others in the care and support of individuals with dementia	**3.1** Explain how to increase a carer's understanding of dementia and a person centred approach See evidence activity 3.2, page 34
	3.2 Demonstrate how to involve carers and others in the support of an individual with dementia See evidence activity 3.2, page 48

3

Communication and Interaction
DEM 205 Understand the factors that can influence communication and interaction with individuals who have dementia

In this unit we look at how communication is fundamental to our sense of 'personhood'. It is a human right and a basic need.

What are you finding out?
We will look at the factors that influence communication and interaction, and how dementia affects the person's ability to verbally communicate. Using a person centred approach we will think about the strengths and abilities of the person with dementia and how we can use their biography to enhance positive interactions.

Reading this unit and completing the activities will allow you to:

• Understand the factors that can influence communication and interaction with individuals who have dementia

• Understand how a person centred approach may be used to encourage positive communication with individuals with dementia

• Understand the factors which can affect interactions with individuals with dementia

LO1 Understand the factors that can influence communication and interaction with individuals who have dementia

Communication is a very complex process and many communication skills can be lost when someone has dementia. However, we must not exclude people with dementia or discriminate against them when we are communicating, just because it might be more difficult for them to understand us, or for us to make ourselves understood. We will discover that people with dementia may not always be able to communicate verbally and may rely on other means of communication and so it is important to understand the different ways in which we interact with each other.

We must understand other difficulties faced by the person with dementia. Not only are their communication skills affected, they also may not be able to recognise previously familiar people or places. If this is the case they will not be able to **interact** with them in the same way as before. Part of our role is to support family members in their interaction with the person with dementia. They may need to adapt their conversation or look at other ways of interacting. This might include simple activities like looking at a magazine together, or talking about past times, or listening to music. All of these interactions are valid ways of interacting and communicating.

Information may be misinterpreted which causes people with dementia to behave in ways that are 'odd' or 'challenging' to us.

1.1 How dementia may influence a person's ability to communicate and interact

What do we mean by 'communication'?

Is it just talking and listening?

Communication is a two way process between people – a way of getting our message across. This can be called an interaction because communication is set in social situations. This interaction can be through speech (verbal) or non-verbal methods, including sounds and body language. We have many ways of communicating, not just talking and listening, and it is particularly important to use our varied communication skills

when we are interacting with a person with dementia. Factors that can affect communication for a person with dementia could include the type of dementia a person has, their life experiences (life story) and their environment. Although we know that dementia affects each person differently, there are often similarities in some of the **deficits** they experience.

Key terms

Deficit is a particular loss or lack of a function, often caused by memory loss in dementia.

Communication has a pattern:

The sender. This is the person who starts the communication process by sending the message.

The receiver. Describes the person to whom the message is sent and who 'makes sense' (interprets) the message. We therefore 'take turns' when we communicate.

A person in the early stages of dementia will continue with the 'pattern' but as the dementia progresses the person will have difficulty in following the flow of a conversation and will not necessarily adopt the role of sender or receiver. They will have difficulties making themselves understood. This is called 'expressive communication'.

Feedback. This is the response which tells us whether the message has been received. A response might, for example, include a verbal reply, a nod of the head or a sigh. The response does not necessarily indicate whether the message has been understood, but it is feedback to the sender who can then decide how to respond.

Evidence activity

1.1 Different responses

Think about a situation (an interaction) where you used different responses when you received a message. Are there situations when verbal feedback is unnecessary or inappropriate?

The channel. This refers to the method by which the message is sent (for example a telephone call). For a person with dementia these methods may decrease. They will lose the capacity to manage telephone calls, write letters and so on.

The context. This is the setting or situation in which the communication takes place. This might be a conversation you have in a place, for example a resident's bedroom in a care home **(the setting)** or you are reassuring someone who is very anxious and upset **(the context)**.

Evidence activity

 Communication context

Describe a situation when the context of a situation caused you to communicate in a particular non-verbal way.

Verbal communication. Speaking is the most obvious type of verbal communication. However, we can also include singing, and laughing or any expressive sound a person might make.

Evidence activity

 Verbal communication

Make a list of the different settings and contexts in which you have encountered verbal communication this week. Think about how a person with dementia may have interacted in these situations.

Non-verbal communication includes:

- eye contact
- reading
- writing
- dancing
- gestures
- behaviour.

We use communication constantly, to:

- express and share our emotions
- express and share an opinion
- share and receive information
- entertain and be entertained
- influence others and be influenced.

We know that we use communication to share information and feelings. It helps us to empathise and to support other people. The signals we receive when we communicate influence the way we think, feel and act all the time, in many different ways. Communication is a fundamental part of being a person and individual. It also is a vital part of interaction between people. As communication skills become more limited for the person with dementia, so does their ability to clearly express what they think, feel or need. This means that they are less able to participate in communication and less likely to empathise. They will also be less able to participate in social situations, because they will lose the capacity to understand and manage the 'rules' of interaction. For example, a person with dementia may find difficulty in joining in a conversation with a group of people, or following the rules of a board game or sharing a joke. This inevitably can lead to feelings of isolation and frustration.

Because of the isolation a person with dementia may feel, it is vital that we form person centred relationships with them. It is a sad fact that in a survey in 2007, the Alzheimer's Society found that over the course of six hours a person with dementia in a care home spent only two minutes talking to staff except when they were undertaking personal care tasks. Can you imagine how you would feel?

1.2 Identify other factors that may influence an individual's ability to communicate and interact

Communication is affected by both **negative** and **positive** factors.

Negative factors are sometimes called 'noise'. This describes anything that might interfere in the accurate sending or receiving of a message – the barriers to effective communication. In this section we will explore those barriers.

We can assume that people with dementia are unable to communicate if they cannot verbalise their thoughts. This assumption is a negative factor.

'Everyone I met has been absolutely amazed that I can still talk and think, even though I have a diagnosis of dementia. They do not understand it. I think that is indicative of what the public thinks.'

'Sometimes they think of you as gaga [speaking slowly] ... Can you do this, can you do that?'.

These extracts are taken from the National Dementia Strategy.

In fact the current culture in health and social care promotes **a person centred approach**, which emphasises the uniqueness of the person and recognises that in order to promote wellbeing it is important to communicate effectively with the person with dementia. As we see from the quotes above, people with dementia may lack the opportunity to express themselves because we make assumptions about their dementia rather than seeing the person first and finding ways to communicate.

Barriers which influence communication

Internal factors

The ability of the person to understand verbal and non verbal messages.

External factors

The way the message is delivered (use of empathy, the correct language, the appropriate tone of voice, etc.).

People with dementia often have other problems, including **sensory impairment**. This can add to their communication difficulties. Someone with hearing loss may use a hearing aid or lip read. A person with poor sight will probably rely on spectacles. However, a person with dementia is already struggling to 'make sense' of the world and their lack of sight or hearing complicates this. They may not be able to understand the need for a hearing aid and cannot tolerate one, or may regularly lose their spectacles. They may not be able to see your gestures or hear your explanation. This can lead to greater feelings of isolation and frustration.

Physical discomfort or pain

This affects the **context** in which the message is sent. A person with dementia is just as likely to suffer pain but may not be able to express it in the same way as you or me. They might misinterpret where the pain is, express their emotion with noises rather than speech, or behave differently from usual. Pain can distract people from listening and concentrating and understanding. They may appear agitated or withdrawn.

Anxiety

People with dementia can feel unsafe in their environment, or in the company of people, particularly if it is noisy and there are many distractions. This can lead to anxiety and signs of distress.

It can be difficult to communicate with an anxious person because they can become preoccupied and irritable. They may be trying hard to make sense of their situation rather than giving you their attention.

Sadness (depression)

Communication may be more difficult because the person cannot give **feedback.** Depression affects significant numbers of people with dementia. This depression may lead to apathy and withdrawal, making it very difficult for them to respond to communication.

Anger

Barriers to communication can lead to feelings of frustration and anger in the person with dementia. If communication is difficult the person may feel isolated or 'unheard'. Communication difficulties are distressing and frustrating. Behaviour (including 'behaviour that challenges') is a form of communication and should not be dismissed as awkward or difficult. Instead it is important to look for the feelings behind the behaviour and not rely on stereotypical assumptions or assume the use of antipsychotic medication will help this behaviour.

English as a second language

We must not assume that everyone we support will use English as their first language. Cultural and language differences must be acknowledged and respected and not seen as barriers. The correct **medium** (the way in which the message is delivered) must be found.

Noise levels

Some of us live or work in noisy environments which can distract or overstimulate a person with dementia. Communication is affected when there are too many signals or pieces of information coming in at once. Remember, for the person with dementia living in a care home, the noise level may be constantly too high and they may not be able to communicate their need for space and silence unless you support them in making those choices. Life stories can help too because by finding out about someone's past life and personal preferences, you may find that they do not like to be in a noisy place.

Environment

We know that a person with dementia may rely on non-verbal types of communication. This might include signage, pictures, colour coding and other visual clues. An environment that is unhelpful in this way can increase a person's level of dependence as well as emphasise their disability. This is called the '**Social Model of Disability**'.

Pressures – from time, other people

We might be supporting people with dementia in collective care settings like care homes or day centres, or visiting people in their own home in the community. We will all work to a schedule, whatever the environment. We will be expected to take responsibility for ourselves and manage our workload. This routine does not always effectively support communication unless we remember to put the person first and ensure we have an understanding of the best way of communicating with them. Rushing can be counterproductive – the message is not received because it has been sent too quickly. The result can be frustration on both sides and a breakdown in communication.

Case Study

  Gladys

Gladys has advanced dementia. She lives in a care home. She is very settled, but staff do not spend very much time with her because she does not seem to need a lot of attention. She spends a lot of her day winding wool and humming. The new manager observes the lack of staff intervention with Gladys.

1) Discuss with your manager or a colleague the issues that the manager might raise with staff.

2) How can she encourage person centred communication with Gladys?

Our own emotions

The way we are feeling affects the **context** in which we communicate. It is important that we have feelings of 'wellbeing' and that we are confident with our communication skills. If we do not understand how it might feel for the person with dementia we will find it hard to communicate using empathy and this can create **barriers**. We

must learn to respond to emotions rather than just the words. If we are impatient or lacking in empathy we are creating barriers.

1.3 How does memory impairment affect the ability of an individual with dementia to use verbal language?

Generally, dementia affects short-term memory first. We rely on our short-term memory to learn and then retain new information. For instance, we learn new words and retain them. We are introduced to a person for the first time and we remember their name because we can use our short-term memory. This is very difficult and eventually impossible for the person with dementia. They forget the words and cannot relearn them because they cannot access their short-term memory. Generally, it is the automatic language skills – responses like 'hello' which are said without thinking which we keep the longest. Those parts of communication that require more complicated or sophisticated thought are lost sooner. Reading and writing become difficult and eventually impossible because the written word has no meaning.

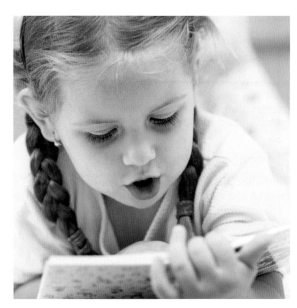

Figure 3.1 As we develop we learn and retain new words. This skill is impaired by the process of dementia.

Difficulties encountered include:

- forgetting names
- forgetting the meaning of words
- using inappropriate words
- substituting words for one with a similar meaning
- replacing the word with a similar sounding one
- describing an object rather than naming it.

The word used to describe these difficulties is **dysphasia**.

The time line below describes a sequence of events. This sequence will not be the same for every person with dementia, but the time line does help us understand the **progressive** effect dementia has on verbal communication skills.

Time →

The person with dementia loses the ability to think of the right word

knowing when to reply

topics of conversation become more limited

the person is unable to explain their own thoughts or insights

the person talks about things only related to themself

they are unable to pick up subtle messages, humour or sarcasm (they may struggle to interpret common colloquial sayings like 'when hell freezes over')

the person speaks less and conversation is more repetitive and routine, only everyday words are used

the person cannot keep to the topic being discussed

conversation becomes vague and rambling

the person makes less and less sense

words and sentences are repeated

it becomes very difficult to put sentences together

only everyday words might be used

the person struggles to pronounce letters and words

the person may stop talking or keep repeating a particular word or phrase or noise.

Figure 3.2 Communication time line.

LO2 Understand how a person centred approach may be used to encourage positive communication with individuals with dementia

In Chapter 2 we learnt about a person centred approach to dementia. This is based on each person being unique, on putting the person at the centre of all our interaction and remembering 'PERSON first, dementia, second'. We can use this same approach when we communicate with a person with dementia. This is done:

- by identifying their communication strengths and abilities
- adapting our style of communication to meet those strengths, abilities and needs
- looking at how we can use information about the person's preferred method of communication to reinforce their uniqueness.

 Identifying the communication strengths and abilities of an individual with dementia

We have already learnt that we cannot always rely on verbal communication and if we are to understand the communication strengths of the person with dementia we may have to use a variety of methods.

1. **Talk to the person.** Make time to chat. Make sure they are aware you are talking to them by using good eye contact. You may need to

gain their attention by gently touching and calling their name. Think about the type of information you are seeking. What do you want to know – you may not get the answers you expect but be happy to be led by the person.

Keep sentences short and simple, do not overload the person with questions, make statements and stick to one point at a time. Do not ask questions that need a complicated answer, and use body language and tone of voice to illustrate what you are saying.

In the course of the conversation you will have the opportunity to discreetly observe their body language. For example – do they smile at certain things, can they hear better on a particular side, do they like to recite poetry, do they respond better to singing?

2. **Observation**. This is a very important way of understanding any aspect of a person with dementia. In terms of their communication skills, it is better to observe them in a variety of settings and contexts. Observe how they react to you and others in a one-to-one context. How do they react in a group – for example in the dining room? How do they make their wishes known – are they able to demonstrate the choices they want to make? Do they respond better to visual clues, or music, for example?

3. **Talk to family and friends**. Do not underestimate how much a person's family and friends know about them. We will look at this in more detail in the section about life story work. They will be able to explain more about the person's likes and dislikes, their current communication skills and strengths.

4. **Talk to colleagues**. Supporting a person with dementia is often team work. Share information and use this to build a profile and add to the person centred care plan.

Research and investigate 🔍

Research the type of information that you could add to a personal profile or life story that would support the person with dementia with their communication skills.

2.2 How to adapt the style of communication to meet the needs, strengths and abilities of an individual with dementia

We have looked at some different ways of communicating and why it becomes increasingly difficult for the person with dementia to communicate. We will now think about how we can adapt our communication and tailor it to the needs of the person. Bear in mind that due to memory loss the person may think they are meeting you for the first time. Try not to point out such 'mistakes' but rather work on the positive aspects of your interaction with them. When you are communicating with the person, try to minimise excess noise and distractions.

Observation and use of body language, including sign language. Think about how close you are to the person. Try not to invade their personal space or make them feel crowded. People with dementia can misinterpret body language and may feel threatened or frightened if you get too close to them or touch them without first building up a rapport.

Adapting your own style of speech and tone of voice. Avoid talking too quickly or too slowly (talking slowly and deliberately can sound patronising). Avoid extremes – do not talk too loudly as this can feel intimidating or too quietly as the person can feel frustrated trying to hear. Use a warm even tone. If the person becomes agitated do not escalate the situation by raising your voice above theirs. Change tactics and if possible, give them space and offer gentle distraction.

Facial expressions. You can 'read' facial expressions and take a cue from them. A person with little facial expression may not understand what you are communicating to them or they may be depressed and unable to express their emotion. It is very important not to assume that a bland expression has little meaning, but rather you must explore using other means, what is happening for that person. Equally, a person with dementia will look at you, taking clues and cues from the way you respond. One technique is to mirror their expression. For example, if the person looks sad you can copy the facial expression and say 'you seem sad'. This might trigger a response because the person can see their own feeling reflected on your face.

Sensory. Check people have the right spectacles and hearing aids (if they can tolerate them). Make use of the senses – this includes the correct level of lighting, aromatherapy, use of music and sounds like birdsong and touch.

Adapting the environment. Make it more meaningful for the person with dementia. Signage and colour coding will support people with dementia more effectively. They may no longer be able to read signs but may still be able to interpret images, like toilet signs, or differentiate strong primary colours.

Life story work. This helps us to understand the history and profile of the person with dementia. The more we know and understand about the person, the more we can support them in a manner that is person centred and meets their needs.

Validation techniques. These acknowledge the emotional aspect of communication. It seeks out the 'expressed emotion', as well as acknowledging it, and tries to reach and communicate with the person through their emotions. Validation is an appropriate response. If the person says one thing, for example 'I need my mother', do they actually want their mother or do they really want comfort? It does not matter if the statement is not 'true'; it is what the person feels at the time that you must explore.

Research and investigate

  (2.3) Communication and care plans

Look at the communication section in some care plans. Do they describe 'barriers to communication'? How could you improve this part of the care plan?

(2.3) Describe how information about an individual's preferred methods of communication can be used to reinforce their identity and uniqueness

We have looked at person centred care in some detail, and in this section we will continue to understand how this supports communication skills. Getting to know the person also involves paying attention to the way they communicate

---

Case Study

 Mrs Brown

Mrs Brown lives in a care home. She has moderate to severe dementia. She forgets that she is in the care home and sees it rather as her own house, often telling people to 'get out'. She is constantly looking for her purse and accuses the staff and her family of stealing it. In previous years Mrs Brown had worked in a factory as a supervisor. She gets frustrated and angry when staff try to remind her that she can no longer tell people what to do. She tends to talk in short repetitive sentences and finds it difficult to concentrate. She is becoming more agitated and aggressive and the home manager feels that they can no longer meet her needs.

Understand the causes:

- Mrs Brown is worried about her money – it is very important to her because she always struggled to 'make ends meet'.

- She becomes anxious when she does not have her 'work' to do. She is keen to support others and will often find her way to the office in the home.

- She is very house proud.

- It is not possible because of her dementia to have insight into her current situation. In her reality, she is at work and cannot understand why she is being told she does not have a job.

Questions

1) Discuss this situation with your manager or team leader. How could you support colleagues in understanding Mrs Brown's situation?

2) What communication skills could you use to support Mrs Brown and how could the staff improve their rapport with her?

verbally. They may use particular words and phrases associated with their past or culture. It is important we learn the meaning of the words for that person. In the same way we might use body language to mirror the person's expressions; we can also use the same phrases to 'enter into their world'.

Remember to involve the person's family and friends, particularly when the person with dementia might be using words or gestures that you are finding difficult in interpreting. For example, do not assume that if someone is calling for 'Alfie' they are referring to a person. Using your investigative skills you may find out that Alfie was the person's cat and once you know that, you can communicate with them in a more meaningful manner.

People with dementia often occupy a world that is full of memories, and in the middle to later stages of dementia, as short-term memory becomes more impaired, will relate only to the past as that becomes their reality. **Reminiscing** with the person is key to effective communication. Attempting to bring the person 'back' to your reality can be a barrier to communication. The present may have no relevance to them. It is more person centred to use the person's memories as a starting point. Bear in mind that you must be careful in this approach because some memories are painful and there are times when it would be inappropriate to expect the person to talk about a particular memory.

Key terms

To reminisce is to recall past events and use them to stimulate memory, interactions and communication.

Evidence activity

2.3 Reminiscing

Describe some of the key points in a person's life which may be significant in communicating with a person with dementia. What kind of emotions do these memories evoke?

LO3 Understand the factors which can affect interactions with individuals with dementia

In this section we will think about how **a person's history** can **facilitate positive interactions**. We will look at **different techniques** to help these positive interactions, and explain how **others can enhance interaction** with a person with dementia.

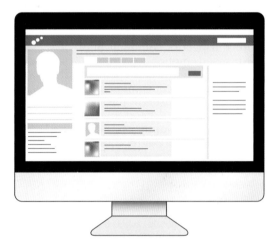

Figure 3.3 We use many ways of communicating and sharing our life experiences.

3.1 Explain how understanding an individual's biography/history can facilitate positive interactions

What do we mean by 'positive interaction'?

We have learnt that communication is a two way process of exchanging messages. Interaction occurs when people are in a situation where they are able to relate to one another and use these social occasions to express and use their social skills.

Any interaction can only be positive if we have some understanding or knowledge of the person we are communicating with. This can vary from simply finding out their name and occupation, or where they live, to something more personal like understanding what frightens them. This knowledge can be the key or trigger to more interaction. It can lead to questions and discovery of things in common, for example. This is no less true for the person with dementia. If we can find out about their personal history, and build a profile of their personhood, we can begin to relate to them because we have the right triggers.

There are different ways of building a personal profile. One of the simplest ways is to use basic questions and use a format that can be kept in the person's room with their life story. Some of the questions you might ask are:

- Where did you grow up?
- What jobs did you do?
- Do you have brothers and sisters?
- What is your favourite food?
- What makes you laugh?

It is important to involve family and friends to help build the profile and to use the questions as your prompts. The person may not wish to answer a question or you may need to re-word it. It should be a 'work in progress' and be used as a positive interaction.

Evidence activity

3.1 Building a personal profile

Prepare a profile for a person you have worked with. Think about what you do and do not know about them. Use person centred questions that will help you learn more about them.

 List different techniques that can be used to facilitate positive interactions with an individual with dementia

Tom Kitwood in his book *Dementia Reconsidered* describes the main psychological needs of a person with dementia as:

- attachment
- love
- comfort
- identity
- occupation
- inclusion.

In order to engage in positive interactions with a person with dementia we must consider the positive and negative aspects of communication. As well as trying to remove the 'barriers' we have discussed we must also understand how we meet a person's psychological needs. Tom Kitwood also talks about positive person work – this means we must strengthen any positive interaction and support it to continue.

In person centred dementia care we **recognise** and **value** the person for who they are. This means treating the person with **respect** and reacting in a way that promotes their **dignity**. Never be dismissive, but rather **listen**. Do not patronise, be **genuine** and recognise that this interaction is one person communicating with another. This means that we **validate** the person's feelings or concerns and respond in ways that give them a **sense of control** or **security**.

Body language is of equal importance.

- Ensure you are on the same level as the person.
- Maintain good eye contact unless it makes them feel uncomfortable.
- Sit or stand in a position where the person can easily see you.
- Mirror their mood and expressions.
- Do not bombard the person with questions but support their conversation and respond to verbal and non verbal clues.
- Use gentle touch to gain attention or reassure.
- Do not invade their personal space or frighten someone by approaching them from behind.
- Go at the person's pace – do not rush them.
- If your face 'doesn't fit' do not persevere. Find a colleague who may get a better outcome or go back later.
- Make sure conversations are about topics enjoyed by the person.

Time to reflect

3.2

Think about Tom Kitwood's description of the six psychological needs. How can you use these to help you to facilitate positive interactions?

For example, in 'attachment', the person with dementia may particularly enjoy holding a particular object because it gives them comfort – they are 'attached' to the object. This might apply to a member of staff or a particular habit like singing as well. Ensure that when you are interacting with them they can maintain that attachment. This could mean you join in the song.

3.3 Explain how involving others may enhance interaction with a person with dementia

We interact with different people in many situations all our life. We all have people in our past and present that are significant to us. It is important for the person with dementia that these personal connections are maintained because we already know that dementia can isolate us from the world. The person with dementia should be enabled to maintain relationships with family and friends – this is called **'relationship centred'** support.

Involving other professionals can also help the person with dementia. It is important to assess the person's needs and then think about those needs that are **'unmet'**. These unmet needs might affect how the person interacts and communicates with others. To address these unmet needs you may need to involve, for example:

- Occupational therapists who can support with appropriate therapeutic activities.
- Activities coordinators who can help engage the person in meaningful activities.
- Speech and language therapists who can support carers in using the right approach.

Evidence activity

3.3 Involving others

Discuss with colleagues and make a list of those professionals who may be able to support people with dementia with positive interactions.

A very helpful website to research is:
www.lifestorynetwork.org.uk

Case Study

   Mrs Jones

Mrs Jones was admitted to a local care home for respite care while her husband was admitted to hospital as an emergency. The staff did not have much information about her because the admission had been very quick. Mrs Jones had moderate dementia. After two hours the care home staff contacted their manager to say that they 'could not cope' because Mrs Jones was trying to leave the building and was 'wandering'.

A nurse from the local mental health team visited the home. She found Mrs Jones alone, walking down a corridor. The nurse spent 30 minutes talking to her and then discussed her conversation with the staff.

As a result of this intervention Mrs Jones settled very quickly. The care home team found her some wool to wind, encouraged her to help with some simple laundry tasks and to socialise with a small group of ladies. They made sure she was kept busy, particularly in the late afternoon.

- What kind of communication skills do you think the nurse used with Mrs Jones in order to find out more about her?
- How do you think she facilitated this positive interaction with her?
- What do you think might form part of Mrs Jones life story that gave the nurse the 'triggers' to work with?

Assessment Summary DEM 205

Reading this unit and completing the activities will have provided you with knowledge, understanding and skills required to understand the factors that can influence communication and interaction with individuals who have dementia.

To achieve the unit, your assessor will require you to:

Learning Outcomes	Assessment Criteria
1 Understand the factors that can influence communication and interaction with individuals who have dementia	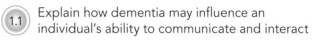 **1.1** Explain how dementia may influence an individual's ability to communicate and interact See evidence activities 1.1, pages 51 and 52
	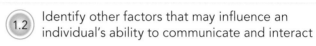 **1.2** Identify other factors that may influence an individual's ability to communicate and interact See case study 1.2, page 54
	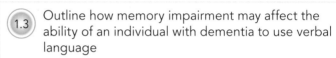 **1.3** Outline how memory impairment may affect the ability of an individual with dementia to use verbal language See evidence activity 1.3, page 55
2 Understand how a person centred approach may be used to encourage positive communication with individuals with dementia	**2.1** Explain how to identify the communication strengths and abilities of a person with dementia See research and investigate activity 2.1, page 56
	2.2 Describe how to adapt the style of communication to meet the needs, strengths and abilities of an individual with dementia See research and investigate activity 2.2, page 57
	2.3 Describe how information about an individual's preferred methods of communication can be used to reinforce their identity and uniqueness See evidence activity 2.3, page 58
3 Understand the factors which can affect interactions with individuals with dementia	**3.1** Explain how understanding an individual's biography/history can facilitate positive interactions See evidence activity 3.1, page 59
	3.2 List different techniques that can be used to facilitate positive interactions with an individual with dementia See time and reflect 3.2, page 60
	3.3 Explain how involving others may enhance interaction with an individual with dementia See evidence activity 3.3, page 60

DEM 210 Understand and enable interaction and communication with individuals with dementia

What are you finding out?

This unit is about communication issues for people with dementia, and how it is important to overcome barriers to communication. We will learn how to gather 'evidence' about the person's preferred methods of communication and how to enhance interaction in a person centred way, using different techniques.

Reading this unit and completing the activities will enable you to:

- Communicate with individuals with dementia

- Apply interaction and communication approaches with individuals with dementia

LO1 Be able to communicate with individuals with dementia

1.1 **Describe how memory impairment can affect the ability of an individual with dementia to use verbal language**

One of the main symptoms of dementia is memory loss. Different parts of the brain are affected which impacts on different aspects of verbal communication. Verbal language is **expressive communication.**

Communication is a two way process – we respond to each other because we understand the rules of exchange. This is not easy for the person with dementia, who may not be able to process language quickly or may not recognise speech patterns. Due to their impairment they may forget names, phrases and sentence construction. We therefore cannot expect them to use the same rules of communication and we must adapt our own methods of communicating.

Unfortunately, impaired verbal communication is immediately noticeable, and this can add to the stigma of dementia. Part of our role as carers is to reduce that stigma by supporting the person to communicate in other ways. We must respond to how they actually are rather than what we expect or assume them to be.

As word finding or remembering becomes more difficult for the person with dementia, the content of their verbal exchanges can become more limited. The person may start to use generalised terms to describe a specific thing or person. For example they may call every male carer 'Fred' because that is the name they have retained.

People with dementia are usually less and less able to retain and use new memories or learning, and so you must be prepared to revisit each situation and conversation as a fresh experience. Words may be forgotten and alternatives found or body language used to help the process.

Memory loss can cause the following problems:

- **Aphasia** – this is when a person has difficulty in processing language – they find difficulty with 'word finding', and eventually putting sentences together. This naturally limits topics of conversation and the person finds difficulty in expressing their thoughts and feelings. Imagine how it must feel if you are unable to tell people what you want or express how you feel.

- **Dysphasia** can affect one or more of aspects of language:
  - comprehension (understanding spoken language)
  - naming (identifying items with words)
  - repetition (repeating words or phrases) and speech
  - expressive dysphasia means that the person finds difficulty in starting a conversation and cannot necessarily put the words in the correct order, or form words.

1.2 **Gather information from others about an individual's preferred methods of communicating to enhance interaction**

As short-term memory fades and the person with dementia finds increasing difficulty in making themselves understood or understanding others, so we must rely on the input of those people who know them best.

We know that life stories and personal profiles help us to get to know the person better. As well as describing important events in the person's life, they can tell us about significant names of people, places and pets. They can tell us about favourite songs or phrases the person may use or recognise. We can relate more effectively to the person with dementia when we understand what is and has been significant in their life.

Communication should be person centred, taking into account the differences between people – their different backgrounds, level of education and life histories as well as different degrees of cognitive ability. This type of information can be gathered from the person themselves and 'significant others' in their life.

1.2 Gathering information from others

Think about a significant person or event in your life. What important information would your family need to tell your carer so that they could communicate with you effectively?

1.3 Use information about the communication abilities and needs of an individual with dementia to enhance interaction

Once you have gained more information about the person you should be able to respond more appropriately to them. Effective communication enhances the quality of life of people with dementia. Information about communication abilities and needs might include:

- Sensory issues. People with dementia may also have problems with hearing or sight. This means that they may rely on other ways of communicating. It is important to know if they are able to communicate using body language, for example, or whether limited sight reduces the impact of using effective body language.

- Having an awareness of the person's preferred first language. We must not assume that everyone we come across will speak English fluently. If English is not the person's first language you may also need to use an interpreter to help you with research. There are professional issues around using family members as interpreters. You may also need to use images, body language and 'talking mats' to help you. This is a pictorial method of supporting communication. Talking mats were developed by researchers and practitioners at the University of Stirling. They can:

  - help people with dementia to choose what they want to do on a day-to-day basis;
  - help people with dementia remember what they have said;
  - provide a structure for conversation between a person with dementia and their family and friends;
  - be used as an activity;
  - help people with dementia to tell family and staff how they feel;

  - provide information for staff about the views of people with dementia;
  - help staff learn more about the person's preferred methods of communication;
  - help staff understand the significance of words, phrases and so on that the person with dementia may use.

- Having an awareness of the personal history and culture of the person with dementia. By being sensitive to the cultural background of the person and their life experiences, you can relate to their use of language and the way they may communicate with you. For example, people may express their thoughts and feelings by referring to their life experiences. The ex-teacher may tell you that you are 'a good girl' or the ex-nurse may want to look after you. It is important to support the person by acknowledging the feelings they are expressing.

1.3 Mrs Smith

Mrs Smith has moderate dementia and has limited speech. She tends to say 'yes' and 'no' or sings songs from the 1950s. She also likes to dance. You can see that she is particularly upset when you are interacting with her. What could you do to support her?

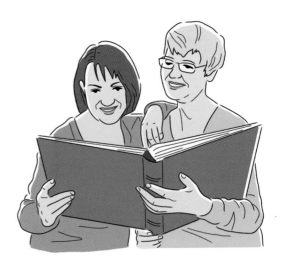

Figure 3.4 Support the person with dementia by communicating in a person centred way.

1.4 Use a person centred approach to enable an individual to use their communication abilities

It is essential for effective communication that it is centred on the person with dementia. Never assume that any person with dementia cannot communicate. It is a matter of working with them to support them in the way that they as individuals are able to communicate.

You must be aware of:

- Barriers to communication for the person – this might include noise, pain and sensory loss.
- Active listening – think carefully about not just what the person is saying but how they say it, their facial expressions, body language and sounds they may make. Do not rely on verbal communication. This is only one aspect of interaction.
- Allowing the person the time to express themselves using their preferred method.
- Not overloading the person with too much stimulation. They may tire easily or become distracted. If necessary, resume the interaction later or use tactile communication, like gentle hand massage to comfort them. Persisting in verbal communication can upset and agitate the person.
- Go at the pace of the person. It will take longer for them to absorb information and to respond. You may need to rephrase. Always be flexible in your approach.
- Be observant. Look for clues about what the person is trying to communicate. For example, it is common for a person to pull at their clothing and walk about in a more agitated way when they need to use the toilet.
- Learn and share. Once you have understood a signal for a particular need or emotion, share that with colleagues. Consistency of approach will support person centred care.

Evidence activity

1.4 Using a person centred approach

Create a table of the different types of communication and how they can support person centred care.

1.5 Demonstrate how interaction is adapted in order to meet the communication needs of an individual with dementia

We know that interaction between people includes verbal and non-verbal communication. As the person with dementia progresses into their dementia 'journey' we may need to rely on more non-verbal methods of communication.

Verbal communication

We cannot assume that the person with dementia will respond verbally in a way we would expect. We have learnt how life stories and personal profiles will help us to talk to the person at their pace and in a context they can relate to. We can adapt our verbal interaction by using a pleasant tone of voice, which is not raised. Shouting can escalate a potentially difficult situation, for example.

We can mirror the person's verbal communication, for example by joining in a song they are enjoying. People with dementia can find it hard to start a conversation. You may need to take the initiative by using familiar words and phrases that are significant and person centred. Remember to attract their attention first by facing them, at eye level, and possibly gently touching them and introducing yourself as they may have forgotten who you are. Use their name and check for reactions.

Here is an example.

Frank is on a ward for people with dementia. He heads for the door. He wants to go to work. The nurse stays with him but does not crowd him. She chats about the day they have had, and does not escalate the situation by dissuading Frank from going to the door. Frank says 'it's cold down here'. The nurse sees the opportunity to use Frank's feelings to support him. 'You are right, Frank, it is cold. Let's go and get warm with a cuppa, I've put the kettle on.'

The nurse adapted her interaction by:

- walking at the right pace with Frank, rather than confronting him
- waiting for an appropriate moment to engage with him rather than impose on him
- listening carefully and taking her cue from Frank, seeing an opportunity to persuade him away from the door by valuing and agreeing with him
- useing a friendly informal approach, with language that Frank relates to.

Non-verbal communication

Body language can be used in a two way process. The person with dementia may express their needs and emotions through their body language and we must learn to understand that language. Equally, we can interact with the person by mirroring them.

Frank approaches the nurse later in the day. He looks very upset. The nurse knows that he finds it difficult to settle in the evenings and often asks for his wife. The nurse adjusts her expression to mirror that of Frank. She says to him 'you look sad, what can I do to help?' Frank says 'is she here?' The nurse starts to talk about Frank's wife and times she knows they spent together. She walks with Frank and he sits. She sits with him and holds his hand.

Although this seems to be a simple interaction, there is actually a lot happening.

Evidence activity

1.5 Adapting interaction

Reflect on this last scenario. List the ways in which the nurse adapted her interaction with Frank. Why is this a person centred approach?

LO2 Be able to apply interaction and communication approaches with individuals with dementia

 List different techniques that can be used to facilitate positive interactions with an individual with dementia

Think about some basic principles first:
- Reduce background noise and distractions.
- Slow your pace.
- Look for non-verbal signs to work out what the person may be feeling.

- Bear in mind that, due to their memory loss, the person may think they are meeting you for the first time.
- Do they respond positively to gentle touch – stroking the back of their hand, for example?
- If the person says one thing, do they mean another? Do they actually mean they want their mother or do they really want comfort and reassurance? What matters is not whether the statement is 'true'; it is what the person thinks or feels at that time. This is what you should respond to.
- Validation is an appropriate response. You might say 'You must miss your mum' and talk about the feelings. Respond to the feelings not the words.
- Do not correct or confront – it rarely helps and it makes people feel devalued.
- Do not worry about tears or laughter – go with the flow.
- Little and often. Do not use long, complicated sentences, and rephrase if necessary.

Remember that you cannot rely solely on verbal communication. Songs, rhymes and sayings might be more relevant to the person. If they are unable to communicate effectively verbally, be imaginative and use all the senses.

- **Sight**. Use images and photographs to stimulate a response. Reminiscence is helpful, looking at reminders of the past and present. Signage that is helpful and body language, smiles and gestures and mirroring can all help.
- **Touch**. Be aware that not everyone responds positively to touch so assess each interaction carefully. It is also important that 'signals' are not misread. However, holding hands, gentle hand massage or a hug when appropriate can be of great comfort and reassurance. People may also respond to touching different materials. Texture can be very meaningful. Think about how you feel when you stroke a pet or touch something cool and smooth.
- **Hearing**. People often have an emotional response to music and poetry.
- **Smell**. Smells can be evocative – think about the smells of baking, or lavender or furniture polish. They can conjure up memories and stimulate a response.
- **Movement**. Activity can be therapeutic. It can range from tapping feet to music, to 'circle dancing'. People with dementia can express themselves and connect with their environment.

2.1 Different techniques for interaction

Explain what might be important things to consider in your approach to ensure that you get a positive response.

 ## 2.2 Use an individual's biography/history to facilitate positive interactions

When we first meet a person, as well as finding out their name, we usually exchange some information with them.

So it is with the person with dementia. In order to facilitate a positive interaction it is your responsibility to take the initiative and learn more about them. In doing so you will be able to empathise and share experiences and feelings.

Evidence activity

2.2 Your life history

Reflect on your first meeting with a friend or colleague. What did you want to know about them? How did you use this information to build your relationship with them?

Talking about someone's history with them can also raise self-esteem, because it makes the most of the ability to remember the past and contributes to a person's sense of identity.

Memorabilia like household objects, certificates of achievements, a favourite possession and so on can be used as 'triggers' to help people with dementia to reminisce.

There are some circumstances when it is particularly important to ensure there is positive interaction with the person with dementia, and where the person's biography and history will support them. These circumstances include admission to hospital or a care home.

Some hospitals and care homes now include person profiles to help this transition. The profile might include:

- My communication strengths and needs (difficulties) are..............................
- For breakfast, lunch and tea I like to eat...
- I like my tea/coffee with.............................
- ....
- I do/don't like television
- I do/don't like a lot of noise around me
- I do/don't sleep well at night
- The name of the person in my photograph is..
- Things that upset me.................................
- ....
- Things that comfort me.............................
- ....

Evidence activity

 2.2 Using a personal profile

How will this profile help positive interaction, particularly with a person with dementia you have just met? What other things could you add to the profile?

2.3 Demonstrate how the identity and uniqueness of an individual has been reinforced by using their preferred methods of interacting and communicating

We are who we are because of our upbringing and networks, our feelings and beliefs. In order to reinforce a person's uniqueness and personhood we must communicate with them in a way that optimises their capacity (makes the most of their ability) to interact and communicate. In this section we have looked at the different elements that help us to understand and enable that interaction in a person centred way.

Memory Impairment. To begin we must have an understanding of how the person's memory impairment affects their ability to communicate.

Information from others about preferred methods. Once we know how communication is affected we can talk to significant others about how the person with dementia prefers to communicate.

Information about communication abilities and needs. With this information we can then begin to adjust our own methods of interaction with the person with dementia.

Person centred approach. To ensure we are person centred, we can use their strengths and needs as our prompts. We must think about communication and interaction from the perspective of the person with dementia

Adapting interaction. We must be creative and think about the most effective ways of communication, knowing the strengths, weaknesses and preferences of the person.

Different techniques. There are many methods of communication at our disposal, including the use of life stories and personal profiles.

Assessment Summary DEM 210

Reading this unit and completing the activities will have provided you with knowledge, understanding and skills required to understand and enable communication and interaction with individuals who have dementia.

To achieve the unit, your assessor will require you to:

Learning Outcomes	Assessment Criteria
1 Be able to communicate with individuals with dementia	**1.1** Describe how memory impairment can affect the ability of an individual with dementia to use verbal language See evidence activity 1.1, page 63
	1.2 Gather information from others about an individual's preferred methods of communicating to enhance interaction See evidence activity 1.2, page 64
	1.3 Use information about the communication abilities and needs of an individual with dementia to enhance interaction See case study 1.3, page 64
	1.4 Use a person centred approach to enable an individual to use their communication abilities See evidence activity 1.4, page 45
	1.5 Demonstrate how interaction is adapted in order to meet the communication needs of an individual with dementia See evidence activity 1.5, page 66
2 Be able to apply interaction and communication approaches with individuals with dementia	**2.1** List different techniques that can be used to facilitate positive interactions with an individual with dementia See evidence activity 2.1, page 67
	2.2 Use an individual's biography/history to facilitate positive interactions See evidence activity 2.2, page 67
	2.3 Demonstrate how the identity and uniqueness of an individual has been reinforced by using their preferred methods of interacting and communicating See evidence activity 2.3, page 68

DEM 308 Understand the role of communication and interactions with individuals who have dementia

What are you finding out?

This unit is about how to understand the role of communication and interactions with individuals who have dementia. In this unit you will understand that people with dementia may communicate in different ways. The unit will explore how individuals with dementia may communicate through behaviours and the impact that this may have on how such behaviour is understood. Difficult, complex and sensitive aspects of communication include issues of a personal nature or distressing situations. The unit provides the underpinning knowledge required to develop therapeutic relationships with individuals with dementia based on interactions and communication.

Reading this unit and completing the activities will enable you to:

- Understand that individuals with dementia may communicate in different ways
- Understand the importance of positive interactions with individuals with dementia
- Understand the factors which can affect interactions and communication of individuals with dementia

LO1 Understand that individuals with dementia may communicate in different ways

1.1 Explain how individuals with dementia may communicate through their behaviour

As a health and social care support worker exchanging information is an important part of your daily routine. Getting to know the people that you support and care for provides you with vital clues to the ways they communicate and how they interact. You will develop many different relationships with individuals with dementia, colleagues and practitioners. Establishing respect for one another can play a significant role in your ability to provide effective care and support.

It is important to note that because dementia is a progressive condition, communication and interactions may fluctuate and will change during the course of every individual's dementia journey. Losing the ability to communicate can be extremely frustrating and difficult for individuals with dementia. As the individual's dementia progresses, the ability to communicate gradually diminishes. Over time it becomes increasingly difficult for individuals to understand what is being said to them, how to understand other people's behaviours and how to express their feelings, needs, wishes and day-to-day conversations.

> ### Key terms
>
> Communication is the activity of conveying meaningful information, there are two forms:
> - verbal
> - non-verbal.

Evidence activity

1.1 Communication

Think about a time when you were on holiday or speaking to someone whose first language was not English. How did that make you feel? What changes did you make to your method of communications?

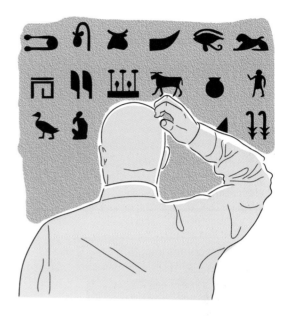

Figure 3.5 Losing the ability to communicate can be extremely frustrating for everyone involved.

1.2 Give examples of how carers and others may misinterpret communication

Communication is the activity of conveying meaningful information. Communication is achieved when the receiving parties understand. For communication to occur there needs to be a place where communications are pooled and interpreted. This is sometimes called communicative commonalty or, put simply, a pot where information is caught and understood. As we have discussed, communication takes various forms:

- verbal communication
- non-verbal communication
- environmental communication.

Carers and others can often misinterpret communication. There a number of reasons why this may happen. The individual with dementia may be finding it difficult to understand information because their brain is not making sense of the information in the same way as it used to.

Problems with communication

In the table below, think about the ways in which communication can be misinterpreted and in some case can lead to labelling individuals in a negative way. Examples could be 'whinging' or kicking off. What terms can you think of that people may use when describing challenges to communication?

Method of communication or interaction	Labels	Explanations
An individual with dementia may repeat what they are saying.		
May take longer to find a word or have difficulty in finding the correct word. These are often the names of objects, places, people.		
Problems in initiating or following conversations.		
Reduced ability to maintain concentration with the television or reading a book or magazine.		
Be forgetful with the topic being discussed.		
The individual may say things that are not true.		
Many of these problems worsen as the person's dementia develops.		
An individual may shout, withdraw or become upset.		
Displaying behaviour that challenges.		

1.3 Explain the importance of effective communication to an individual with dementia

When adopting a person centred approach it is important to consider the person not their dementia. See the person first. It is important to consider whether there are there any other issues or problems that may be causing communication difficulties, for example visual or hearing impairment. Is the environment busy or distracting or perhaps there are cultural differences that may have been overlooked. Always communicate directly with the individual with dementia and not through a third party such as a family member friend or practitioner. Talking about the individual in front of them can make them feel insignificant as information previously unknown to the individual with dementia can be discussed.

Evidence activity

1.3 Explain the importance of effective communication

This activity will show you how you can promote positive interactions and communications.

In the table below list ways that can improve communications and interactions.

How do these techniques improve communication?

Why do they promote positive communication?

	What	How	Why
Staff			
Residents			
Visitors			
Environment			

1.4 Describe how different forms of dementia may affect the way an individual communicates

As discussed in Chapter 1 there are over 100 conditions and diseases that cause dementia. In addition, the chapter showed how Alzheimer's disease could also be compounded by a vascular dementia in order to illustrate how every case of dementia is distinctive. The notion of diversity also addressed individuals as unique because of the different backgrounds people may come from. Therefore it is important to be aware that every person with dementia is unique and the problems experienced in communicating thoughts and feelings and interacting with others are different for all individuals. Language skills can become affected in terms of speaking, receiving and understanding feedback. **Aphasia** is where a person's ability to understand what is being said to them is impaired. In a similar way, reading and writing skills may also deteriorate. **Dysarthia** is the term used to describe a language disorder where speech often becomes unclear.

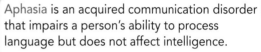

Key terms

Aphasia is an acquired communication disorder that impairs a person's ability to process language but does not affect intelligence.

www.aphasia.org

Dysarthia is difficulty in speaking where speech becomes unclear, often in the case of a stroke.

Some changes in communication

Each person with dementia is unique and the difficulties experienced in communicating thoughts and feelings are different for each individual. There are many causes of dementia, each affecting the brain in different ways.

Some changes you might notice in the person with dementia include:

- They may have difficulty in finding a word. A related word might be given instead of one they cannot remember.
- They may talk fluently, but not make sense.
- They may not be able to understand what you are saying or may only be able to grasp part of it.
- They may lose the normal social conventions of conversation and interrupt or ignore a person.
- They may have difficulty in expressing emotions appropriately.

Research and investigate

1.4 Research and investigate one particular way in which dementia can affect communication. Explain some of the main attributes and how you might help the person with dementia cope with the problems they encounter.

LO2 Understand the importance of positive interactions with individuals with dementia

Give examples of positive interactions with individuals who have dementia

First of all it is useful to make sure that an individual's ability to communicate is not due to such things as dirty glasses or a hearing aid that is not turned on.

Eye contact – It is important to maintain good eye contact with the individual with dementia. It is important that eye contact is level with the individual and not from above as this can infer status or power and be intimidating or scary. Eye contact is a way that shows the person that you are interacting with that you are interested and listening rather than concentrating on what is going on around you. It is also important to remember that eye contact can mean different things to different cultures.

Time – Communications with individuals with dementia should not be rushed as this may make the person feel like they are a problem and not important, or that you do not have any respect for them. In the same way, taking too much time could make people feel uncomfortable and incompetent. It is important to get the balance right, the timings should be appropriate for the purpose of the interaction, taking into account the needs of the individual. Individuals should not be interrupted as this may make them feel like they are not worthy and that their personal interests are not being considered properly. Individuals need to be given enough to time process what you have said to them and to interact with you.

Personal space – Sitting next to someone rather than across a table from them can make some people feel at ease. If appropriate, mirroring the individual's body language can also create a sense of togetherness.

Body language – Body language accounts for over 70 per cent of subconscious interaction and so should be considered when communicating with individuals with dementia. Observing your own body language can support good communication by displaying open and positive body language. This indicates that you are actively engaging and that you do not feel uncomfortable. Equally, as a support worker you will get to know people's behaviours and may notice body language that indicates that some one is upset, anxious, angry or maybe in pain.

Active listening – In your role as support worker you can use active listening techniques. Active listening techniques focus on:

- what is being said verbally
- what tone the person is using
- body language

Phrasing or questioning techniques

How questions or statements are put together and delivered can impact on how communication and interaction is understood. It is important to think about the needs of people when collecting or delivering information so as to reduce any feelings of inadequacy or distress. Below are some examples that you may find useful.

Closed questions – For example 'I'm making a cup of tea, would you like one, Mrs Brown?' A disorientated person need only reply 'Yes' or 'No'. A more complex question would need a longer answer, and cause more confusion.

Open questions – For example 'Tell me about your favourite food, Mrs Brown'. This approach allows you to start up a conversation.

Process questions – For example 'What do you think the nurse was saying, Mrs Brown?' This type of question can give you an indication as to the individual's understanding of the situation. Caution should be observed when using this

Evidence activity

2.1 Creating positive interactions

You have taken Mrs Brown out to the park for the morning. It was a lovely crisp and sunny winter's morning and you saw squirrels and fed the ducks. You also watched a group of people playing softball in the park and Mrs Brown loved to watch the game and join in with the excited crowd who cheered. It is cold outside so you decide to go for a cup of tea and some cake in a tea room by the park which overlooks the duck pond.

How could you start a conversation with Mrs Brown?

What forms of questions could you use?

What signs could you look for when communicating with Mrs Brown?

Why would the visual prompt of the duck pond be useful?

technique with individuals in the latter stages of dementia.

Clarification – For example 'I think you said that this made you feel scared. Is that right, Mrs Brown?' This is a useful way of checking or evaluating the outcome of your conversations. This technique also shows that you were actively listening.

Explain how positive interactions with individuals who have dementia can contribute to their wellbeing

The relationships that exist between colleagues, individuals with dementia, their families and friends and practitioners have a huge impact on the quality of care and support that is delivered. Relationships are built on the ways in which way we interact with one another and those around us. Clear, consistent and respectful interactions can assist in promoting wellbeing by considering the perspective of individuals with dementia, because this shows that you respect their cultural background and have a real interest in who they are. By using good communication techniques you will take into consideration any other concerns that may hinder an individual's ability to listen, observe or touch. By taking issues such as these into consideration you will create a comfortable environment for individuals with dementia to communicate effectively. It is important to consider the ways in which the environment may affect spatial awareness and orientation. In essence, how does the environment communicate with individuals with dementia? Pictorial signage, colour contrasts, large clocks, seasonal calendars and good lighting can assist in providing a good environment for communicating and understanding needs. The ways in which the environment communicates assists individuals in understanding what is happening around them. This is called spatial and time orientation. It is common for some individuals with dementia to lose awareness of time. Spatial orientation involves judging distance, height or position of the self in relation to other objects. Through adopting positive communications and interactions individuals feel included and respected and their wellbeing could improve.

Explain the importance of involving individuals with dementia in a range of activities

It is important to involve individuals with dementia in a range of activities because of the ways in which this can provide opportunities for social engagement, engaging with skill sets and increasing senses of wellbeing. Individuals with dementia can often feel isolated as their condition progresses and their communication skills deteriorate. By being involved in activities this kind of inclusive practice can promote a sense of belonging, provide opportunities for rehabilitation and a sense of wellbeing. Activities can range from something that may occur on an everyday basis, such as eating and drinking, to a set of activities based on pursued hobbies or leisure interests. This type of activity can also provide valuable opportunities for getting to know what individuals like to do, what interests them and what things they may like to do in the future. Activities are also a positive way of encouraging individuals to work in groups or on their own. According to the Department of

Case Study

2.2 Harry

Harry has just moved into a care home. He is getting used to the new routine and in the first few days his key support worker has been showing him around the facilities. He is in a wheelchair, is deaf in his left ear and sometimes experiences asphasia. Harry enjoys meeting new people and finding out about what they do. His support worker takes him first to the laundry and then to the kitchen. As Harry loves gardening he asks to go outside to meet the gardener.

- How should Harry be introduced to staff?
- Where and at what level should the support work be in relation to Harry?
- What techniques should Harry's support worker use to promote positive interactions?
- List five ways in which these will improve communication and interactions.

Health there are five main keys to successful involvement, these are:

- accessible information that explains how to be involved
- information that states clearly what the options are
- liberty and freedom to express wishes and wishes
- being listened to, understood and having needs and views respected and heard
- being able to influence what happens and make decisions that matter.

The **social environment** can provide interactions which create stimulation and enjoyment such as:

- opportunities to meet with family and friends.
- being able to talk about early life, past career, good memories
- engagement with familiar activities such as attendance at church, clubs, playing golf, favourite walks
- engagement with activities such as reminiscence, listening to favourite music, reading, art
- continuing social routines, such as going to the hairdressers, out for coffee and so on.

Evidence activity

 Chiwila

Chiwila is a Polish woman with dementia. She speaks very little English and as she progresses through the dementia journey she is reverting more and more to Polish. How can you help Chiwila integrate? How can you get to know what Chiwila likes and dislikes? What kind of activities could you plan for Chiwila?

2.4 Compare a reality orientation approach to interactions with a validation approach

In this section a reality orientation approach will be compared with a validation approach. First, it is important to understand what the concepts mean through definitions.

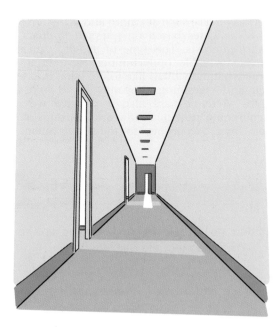
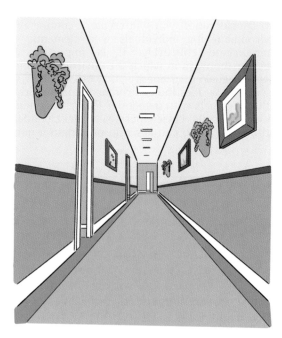

Figure 3.6 The right environment can provide opportunities which create stimulation and enjoyment.

Validation approach

The **validation approach** is based on a general principle of validation. It was developed by Naomi Feil in 1982. The validation approach accepts the perception and reality of another person's experience. As a health and social care support worker you will be using non-judgemental acceptance and empathy to show the individual with dementia that their expressed feelings are valid. A validation approach focuses on the feelings of the individual rather than the content or context of speech. In other words, understanding the feelings behind the subject matter discussed rather than what is said.

For more details see **www.vfvalidation.org**

Reality orientation

Reality orientation has been defined as an approach which may improve confusion and decrease behaviour we find challenging with individuals with dementia. It was developed in the United States in the 1950s. There is not an agreed method of how reality orientation should be communicated but it is generally delivered in the following two ways. First, through constantly orientating individuals in time, place and person on a 24-hour basis and, second, orientating people to reality within a group setting. A reality orientation approach tries to place the individual in the here and now, reminding them of the day, place, time and situation they are in.

Key terms

Validation approach is using non-judgemental acceptance and empathy to show the individual that their expressed feelings are valid. Focusing on the feelings rather than the content of speech.

Reality orientation is an approach that tries to place the individual in the here and now, reminding them of the day, place, time and situation they are in.

Benefits

Reality orientation appeals to existing abilities and aims to promote and rehabilitate skill sets that remain. It uses a series of non pharmacological interventions such as signposts, notices and other memory aids to remind individuals where they are in time and space. Bleathman and Morton (1988) found that verbal skills were improved and extended using this approach.

The validation approach takes into account the emotion behind why, for example, an individual may be expressing that they are looking for their mother who died over 30 years ago. Rather than correcting the individual who is seeking their dead mother by saying that their mother is dead and that they shouldn't ask such questions this approach considers an alternative response that would respond to the emotional drive in someone to look for their mother. With the validation approach you try to rephrase what is said and try to tap into the visual sense with a response such as 'you must miss your mum a lot, what colour hair did she have?', this then provides the opportunity to reminisce and confirm that you have listened and taken the individual seriously.

Limitations

Reality orientation has been described as detrimental to the wellbeing of individuals with dementia due to the fact that the behavioural conditioning serves to remind them of mental and physical deterioration (Goudie and Stokes, 1989) and can lower mood.

Evidence activity

 2.4 Pros and cons

Consider the benefits and limitations of a reality orientation approach and list them down. Now list the benefits and limitations of the validation approach. Think about your work environment and write a short presentation to give to your colleagues during a break.

LO3 Understand the factors which can affect interactions and communication of individuals with dementia

3.1 List the physical and mental health needs that may need to be considered when communicating with an individual with dementia

Physical needs

An individual with dementia may have physical needs such as needing support due to visual impairment, administering medication, appropriate nutrition and hydration (eating and drinking), mobility (walking and transferring), support with personal care, communication and managing pain.

Mental health needs

Mental health is not mental illness. Mental health is about emotional wellbeing and is about feeling positive about who we are and what we feel. Our mental health consists of what makes us who we are; our thoughts, beliefs, values, hopes, fears and our life experiences. Mental health can be affected by internal thought processes and external factors such as the environment and relationships. Of course, it is natural to have good days and bad days – good mental health allows us to balance these out and cope with the emotional spectrum of the ups and downs of everyday life. People with poor mental health take longer to recover from negative life events. Individuals with dementia still have mental health which can benefit from participating in meaningful activities and interactions.

Depression

Statistically, individuals with living with dementia are more likely to become depressed. It is not a given that people with dementia will become depressed, however, and evidence from a large-scale study into mental health and wellbeing found that five key areas can be useful in promoting wellbeing and benefit mental health:

- not experiencing discrimination
- being presented with opportunities to participate in meaningful activities
- positive social relationships
- good physical health
- having enough money.

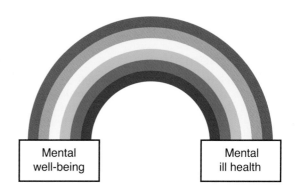

Figure 3.7 Mental health is a spectrum we all experience. We can all suffer mental ill health at times when we feel sad or lonely, but we can also experience happiness and comfort.

Evidence activity

 3.1 **Understand the factors which can affect interactions and communication of individuals with dementia**

In the table below list the barriers that you may have experienced or encountered with other staff, individuals with dementia, families and friends. Are these physical or social barriers? What could you do to improve communication to negotiate the barriers?

Staff	Individuals with dementia	Family and friends	Physical and social environment	Why are these important?	What can be done to improve communication?

3.2 Describe how the sensory impairment of an individual with dementia may affect their communication skills

Some older people may have difficulty communicating because of poor eyesight or hearing. You can assist individuals who have a visual impairment by ensuring they have regular eyesight tests and that their glasses are clean and worn properly. It also helps to make sure that their belongings are kept in the same place. This can assist individuals being able to orientate around the building, recognise people and be able to find their belongings or important items. It could be useful to learn the correct way to guide and assist a partially sighted individual and research what visual aids your organisation has. Individuals with visual impairments may benefit from large print books, menus, talking books and other documents. They might otherwise find it difficult to access information and may socially withdraw. When communicating with visually impaired individuals with dementia it is important that you:

- let them know that you are close in a quiet and calm manner
- introduce yourself by name
- use appropriate forms of touch to start and continue conversation
- ask what form of communication suits them.
- allow the individual to take your arm before leading them around
- treat the individual as unique and do not assume that all visually impaired people have the same communication needs.

You can support individuals with dementia with a hearing impairment by making sure their hearing is tested regularly and that the hearing aid is clean, working and turned on. It also might be useful to learn how to change a hearing aid battery or even how to perform sign language. There may be other aids that you could use too, such as flashing lights instead of telephone ringtones or doorbells. When communicating with individuals with dementia with hearing impairments:

- speak clearly, listen carefully and respond to what is being said
- minimise any distractions such as noisy televisions
- make sure any aids to hearing are working
- use written forms of communications that are appropriate
- use signing where appropriate, by involving a properly trained interpreter.

Key terms

Hearing loop this provides information on an induction loop system, to assist the hearing impaired by transmitting sound from a sound system, microphone, television or other source, directly to a hearing aid.

Time to reflect

3.2 Improving communication

Think about what you can do to improve your communication methods with individuals with dementia who are:

1. partially sighted
2. have a hearing impairment.

What equipment or resources could you use? What new skill set could help you improve? How would this benefit the people you work with?

3.3 Describe how the environment might affect an individual with dementia

The environment can play a pivotal role in how an individual with dementia feels they can communicate. The term 'environment' can be split into two spheres: the social environment and the physical environment.

Physical

The physical environment can be improved to promote positive communication in a number of ways.

Personal space – bedroom

An individual's bedroom is their space, it is a place where they may have friends and family to visit, it is also a place where specialist interventions can take place. Most importantly it is a room that is theirs, therefore it is a space that should convey who they are and what makes them feel a sense of wellbeing. A sign on the door should state clearly their preferred name and use an image that is important to the individual. This not only facilitates orientation and a sense of ownership but also provides visitors with an initial communication subject that is essentially about the individual with dementia. If it is possible, familiar furniture and soft furnishings can create a sense of homeliness. Photographs and memorabilia can personalise a room and when combined with life story work can provide rich communication tools that can prompt conversations that are person centred. This is because the person and their interests and achievements will be at the centre of communications derived from the objects, pictures, photographs, memorabilia and so on that are meaningful. Take a moment to look around the room or at any objects such as jewellery or a phone that you carry on your person. Now think about the different stories you could tell about how you acquired all the objects that you own. Who were you with? Was it a happy time? Does it evoke memories of smelling freshly cut grass? Do you remember anyone in particular? Just by looking at one item you will have probably reminisced about a number of things. This is because social relationships are embedded within the physical environment.

Communal areas

Communal areas are often quite busy and noisy places which can be distracting and overwhelming. This can cause individuals with dementia to exhibit behaviours that demonstrate their discomfort or individuals may socially withdraw. Reducing background noise can provide a more soothing environment where individuals feel that they can be heard and communicate. Sitting rooms can be a more inviting space if chairs and sofas are placed so that interactions can take place or so that individuals can find a quiet place should they choose to. The propensity to place chairs around the outside of a room provides little room for meaningful interactions, rather it presents opportunities where conflict can occur. Televisions can be a useful form of media that individuals can enjoy, however the television should not be on all day and night as an activity. Conflicting media such as the television and music can be very confusing, instead one activity at a time used in a controlled and timely manner can provide impetus for conversations. Pictures used to decorate the walls can also be used to generate meaningful interactions. Gather information about the local area, local occupations and individual's life histories and try to find pictures or local crafts that can be used to enhance your physical environment. The traditional approach to adorning walls is usually finished with elaborate pictures of flowers or unrelated landscapes that have no meaning to anyone and therefore do not promote an inclusive environment. Pictures and objects can be used in a variety of ways to:

- enhance the environment by being inclusive and accessible
- promote senses of belonging and ownership
- provide stimuli for meaningful conversations and interactions
- use as distraction tools.

Social environment

The social environment can provide interactions which create stimulation and enjoyment for example:

- opportunities to meet with family and friends
- ability to talk about early life, past career, good memories
- engagement with familiar activities, such as attendance at church, clubs, playing golf, favourite walks
- engagement with activities, such as reminiscence, listening to favourite music
- continuing social routines, such as going to the hairdressers, out for coffee and so on.

Evidence activity

(3.3) Improving environments

Think about the different areas of your work setting. How does the current environment affect communications? How could you improve this? Write down five ways of improving your environment for each area of your work setting.

 Describe how the behaviour of carers or others might affect an individual with dementia

The behaviours of people who care for and support individuals with dementia can have a significant impact on the person. Carers can often become frustrated or angry in some situations, which can trigger negative feelings and memories. Stress can be very infectious. On the flip side, the behaviour of carers can also be very positive.

Creating a relaxing environment that is free of clutter and that only has things that you need on view can help. Carers have a tendency to overdo things or compensate for perceived lack of abilities. Instead the individual with dementia should be encouraged to continue doing things for themselves such as washing, dressing, tying shoe laces, eating at the dinner table with others, walking and being as active as possible. Activities like joint exercise, such as going for a walk, could assist in promoting a relaxed state and improved sleep patterns. Carers can often find themselves having conversations about the person they are caring for. This can exclude the individual with dementia. Instead, include the individual with dementia in the conversation so that their thoughts and feelings can be considered.

Evidence activity

 Behaviours of carers or others that might affect an individual with dementia

List five ways that the behaviours of carers can affect an individual with dementia:

Positively

1.

2.

3.

4.

5.

Negatively

1.

2.

3.

4.

5.

3.5 Explain how the use of language can hinder positive interactions and communication

It is important to consider how the use of language may hinder positive communication and interactions. Language accounts for only a small percentage of how we communicate but here are some examples of how language can hinder the communication process:

- **Dominance** – if someone dominates the communication process, communication becomes one way and responses from the other person are hindered.
- **Inappropriate self-disclosure** – this is where someone talks too much about themselves.
- **Swearing** – foul language may be perceived to be powerful but it usually turns others off.
- **Jargon** – people often use words that belong to their area of expertise.
- **Patronising** – condescending words, tones or behaviour may make individuals and their families feel angry or defensive.

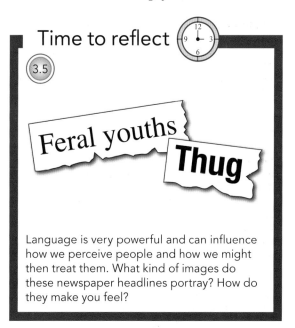

Time to reflect

3.5

Feral youths

Thug

Language is very powerful and can influence how we perceive people and how we might then treat them. What kind of images do these newspaper headlines portray? How do they make you feel?

Assessment Summary DEM 308

Reading this unit and completing of the activities will have provided you with knowledge, understanding and skills required to understand and enable interaction and communication with individuals who have dementia.

To achieve the unit, your assessor will require you to:

Learning Outcomes	Assessment Criteria
1 Understand that individuals with dementia may communicate in different ways	**1.1** Explain how individuals with dementia may communicate through their behaviour See evidence activity 1.1, page 71
	1.2 Give examples of how **carers** and **others** may misinterpret communication See evidence activity 1.2, page 71
	1.3 Explain the importance of effective communication to an individual with dementia See evidence activity 1.3, page 73
	1.4 Describe how different forms of dementia may affect the way an individual communicates See research and investigate 1.4, page 73
2 Understand the importance of positive interactions with individuals with dementia	**2.1** Give examples of positive interactions with individuals who have dementia See evidence activity 2.1, page 74
	2.2 Explain how positive interactions with individuals who have dementia can contribute to their wellbeing See case study 2.2, page 75
	2.3 Explain the importance of involving individuals with dementia in a range of activities See evidence activity 2.3, page 76
	2.4 Compare a reality orientation approach to interactions with a validation approach See evidence activity 2.4, page 77

Learning Outcomes	Assessment Criteria
3 Understand the factors which can affect interactions and communication of individuals with dementia	**3.1** List the physical and mental health needs that may need to be considered when communicating with an individual with dementia See evidence activity 3.1, page 78
	3.2 Describe how the sensory impairment of an individual with dementia may affect their communication skills See time to reflect 3.2, page 79
	3.3 Describe how the environment might affect an individual with dementia See evidence activity 3.3, page 80
	3.4 Describe how the behaviour of carers or others might affect an individual with dementia See evidence activity 3.4, page 81
	3.5 Explain how the use of language can hinder positive interactions and communication See time to reflect 3.5, page 81

DEM 312 Understand and enable interaction and communication with individuals who have dementia

What are you finding out?

In this unit we will further explore the factors affecting communication and how to use positive interaction and care planning. You should be able to develop and implement the qualities of an effective relationship with individuals with dementia.

Reading this unit and completing the activities will enable you to:

• Understand the factors that can affect interactions and communication of individuals with dementia

• Communicate with an individual with dementia using a range of verbal and non-verbal techniques

• Communicate positively with an individual who has dementia by valuing their individuality

• Use positive interaction approaches with individuals with dementia

LO1 Understand the factors that can affect interactions and communication of individuals with dementia

1.1 Explain how different forms of dementia may affect the way an individual communicates

Alzheimer's disease. People in the early stages of Alzheimer's disease may have lapses of memory and have problems finding the right words. As the disease progresses, they become more confused and frequently forget the names of people, places, appointments and recent events. This may inhibit interaction and the person may become withdrawn or depressed because they are unable to interact as well as before. Depending on the reactions of others, if they are unsupported, they can retreat into a shell.

Vascular dementia. People who experience this type of dementia have difficulty concentrating, and communicating. They tend to make visual 'mistakes' and can misperceive – this means they tend to misinterpret their environment or circumstances. This can make interaction more difficult as the person may only have a sense of their own reality and are unable to make sense of yours.

Dementia with Lewy bodies. People with DLB often experience hallucinations which affects their ability to communicate effectively. Their condition also tends to fluctuate so communication and interaction can be inconsistent and unpredictable in its manner and content.

Fronto temporal dementia (including Pick's disease). People may experience language difficulties, including:

- problems finding the right words
- inability to start a conversation or be spontaneous
- using many words to describe something simple
- a reduction in or lack of speech.

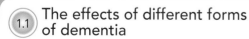

Evidence activity

1.1 The effects of different forms of dementia

Consider the problems a person with fronto temporal dementia may experience. How do they impact on their communication skills and what might the emotional impact of this be?

1.2 Explain how physical and mental factors may need to be considered when communicating with an individual with dementia

We must not assume that it is only their dementia affecting a person's ability to communicate and interact. This is the case particularly for older people who are likely to experience other physical problems. Such problems include poor sight and hearing. The person may also experience pain and discomfort. These factors impede communication. The person may not only struggle to see or hear you, they may find difficulty concentrating because of their pain, or difficulty in speaking because of ill-fitting dentures. Medication may also be a factor – too much or too little medication, or taking incorrect medication should also be considered if the person is having difficulty communicating.

The way we interact and communicate is coloured by our own mental health. The person who is withdrawn or depressed may have more difficulty in starting a conversation, or showing interest in the world around them or keeping up with interactions. It is important to consider whether the person with dementia is also depressed or whether they are unwell with a delirium. Delirium, as we know, can make people more confused or withdrawn.

Case Study

1.2 Mrs Williams

Mrs Williams has poor sight and is in pain from her arthritis. She finds it difficult to concentrate for long. She has Alzheimer's disease. Explain how these factors may affect her communication and interaction with others.

1.3 Describe how to support different communication abilities and needs of an individual with dementia who has a sensory impairment

A person with sensory impairment will usually try to compensate for that loss in some way, but for the person with dementia this can be more difficult. It is important that you work with the person to overcome as many of these barriers as possible and to understand their alternative communication strategies.

Case Study

1.3 Mrs Brown

Mrs Brown has dementia and has hearing loss. She is able to see and understand body language because she has been deaf for some time and has learnt how to cope with that. It is even more important now that carers make best use of that skill, using facial expressions, touch, gestures, pictures and images. You must also consider her most favoured use of communication and not assume because she is deaf she will read lips or understand sign language. One significant problem for her is that she finds difficulty interacting in a group, for example singing or talking and can become withdrawn.

How could you support Mrs Brown to participate in the group?

Case Study

1.3 Mrs Green

Mrs Green has dementia and has poor sight. She enjoys listening to her favourite songs but gets very anxious and agitated if a person talks to her without introducing themselves. She is particularly anxious and challenging when supported with personal care.

What strategies could you use when helping Mrs Green with her care needs?

How should we approach a person when supporting them with personal tasks?

How do we maintain their dignity?

Time to reflect

1.3 Mrs Brown

Mrs Brown has dementia and has poor sight and hearing loss. Imagine what the world must be like for Mrs Brown. She is isolated because she cannot see body language and facial expressions clearly and she cannot really hear when carers try to talk and reassure her. Carers have to rely more on her other senses to help her communicate and interact. They must show great empathy and be clear and consistent with each other about what they understand about Mrs Brown. Think about Mrs Brown's skills – what she is able to do rather than not do?

1.4 Describe the impact the behaviour of carers and others may have on an individual with dementia

We describe carers as partners, family, friends and neighbours. 'Others' might include professionals like the GP or nurse or support groups.

We have learnt that communication and interaction are affected by dementia. It is important that those people who are part of the person's network have a clear understanding of their needs. Refer back to **Unit 308, 3.4** (page 80) for more information.

Carer education and staff training will help in this situation. Family and friends will remember how the person with dementia used to interact and may find the changes in their behaviour frustrating and even embarrassing. It is important to support carers in understanding the reasons for the behaviour and the best ways to interact and react.

A lack of understanding can have a negative impact. Carers may try to 'talk over' the person, finish sentences for them or overcompensate for the person's lack of communication skills. It is all too easy to talk about the person when they are in the same room, forgetting that they have the right to be consulted and included.

Carers should be supported to observe and accept the way the person interacts. Ignoring the messages of body language or dismissing the use of noises and facial expressions is rejecting the individuality of the person. Imagine how you would feel if you thought you were communicating clearly only to find that you are being ignored or your wishes not taken into account.

Equally, when the person with dementia is accepted for who they are and the people around them ensure that they enter into a different world of communication a connection can be made. This is the difference between negative and positive interactions. Tom Kitwood describes interactions and the impact they have in the following ways:

- **Recognition** – interacting in a way that is free from stigma, seeing the person with dementia in their own right.
- **Negotiation** – assumptions are not made about the person and they are consulted with.
- **Collaboration** – the carer does not exert power but gives the person with dementia space to express themselves.
- **Play** – the carer is able to interact in a way that is creative.
- **Timalation** – the person with dementia gains pleasure from their senses.
- **Celebration** – the carer is able to enjoy life with the person with dementia.
- **Validation** – the carer does not use their own terms of reference, but empathises with the person with dementia.
- **Relaxation** – the carer is able to stop and slow down and go at the pace of the person with dementia.
- **Holding** – the carer is able to stand firm and support the person with dementia no matter how emotional or agitated they might be.
- **Facilitation** – a readiness to respond to the gestures the person with dementia makes, sharing in the creation of meaning.
- **Creation** – (by the person with dementia) is acknowledged and responded to. The person with dementia is in control.
- **Giving** – (on the part of the person with dementia). The carer accepts the gifts or gestures of kindness as a real part of the relationship.

Tom Kitwood *Dementia Reconsidered* 1997

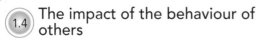

Evidence activity

1.4 The impact of the behaviour of others

Describe one example of a positive interaction with a person with dementia, and one negative example.

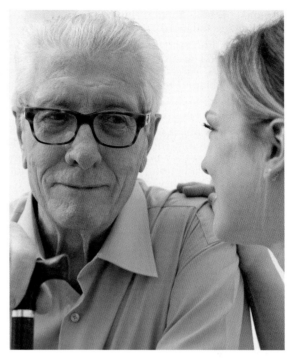

Figure 3.9 Remember that you need to use empathy and 'walk in the shoes' of the person so you can see the world from their perspective and support them appropriately.

LO2 Be able to communicate with an individual with dementia using a range of verbal and non-verbal techniques

2.1 Demonstrate how to use different communication techniques with an individual who has dementia

There are many techniques that will support the various communication needs of the person, using the different senses.

Life story and reminiscences. The person with dementia may communicate using their long-term memories as the present is no longer a reality for them. The use of memorabilia can stimulate positive feelings and encourage the person to share experiences. We have much in common, schooldays, holidays, work and so on, and using these triggers can help us find common ground to talk about. This in turn leads to empathetic exchanges.

Validation. Focusing on the reality of the person with dementia is integral to a person centred approach to care. Validating this reality is particularly helpful when the person is:

- experiencing strong feelings – acknowledge the feeling and treat the person with dignity
- convinced about what they believe to be true – contradicting the person can cause more anxiety and they may not be able to accept that contradiction because they cannot retain your reality
- being given factual information that is not helping the person to feel any better. The most common example is the person who is looking for their mother and they are told that she has died. Imagine how it must feel to be told your mother is dead again and again because you cannot retain that information.

Reality orientation. This is a technique when the person with dementia is supported and reminded to help them understand where they are, what time of day it is and so on. The use of newspapers, prompts about mealtimes, calendars and lists can all help. There is an argument that this technique is not helpful in the later stages of dementia.

Singing and dancing. This might play to the strengths of the person with dementia. Such activities are often retained in memory and can be used not only as a way of social interaction but also to communicate feelings.

Snoezelen. A quiet room designed to stimulate the senses. The Snoezelen may have soft lighting, interesting fabrics and comfortable chairs. There could be soothing music or sounds like birdsong and moving images. This should be used with caution as some people are overwhelmed by the variety of sensory input.

Evidence activity

 2.1 Demonstrate how to use different communication techniques

Think about how you would respond in the following situation, using different communication techniques:

- The person feels lost because they don't know where they are.
- The person is anxious because they don't know who you are.
- The person has misunderstood what's going on.

2.2 Show how observation of behaviour is an effective tool in interpreting the needs of an individual with dementia

When verbal communication is limited and the person with dementia has to rely on their body language and behaviour, we must be more observant. In the normal course of any conversation we use body language more than we realise. We use eye contact and hand signals, for example, and we can express how we feel just by folding our arms. In the case of a person with dementia we need to fine tune our attention and be aware of their behaviour and body language.

There are common misconceptions about the behaviour of a person with dementia and all too often their behaviour can be described as 'challenging'. This might be the case in some instances but it is not true that everyone with dementia displays such behaviour. It is our job to understand the reasons behind the behaviour.

The person may be:

- expressing a wish or an emotion. For example, repeatedly going into the kitchen or dining room may mean the person is hungry or they are unsure of the time of day
- seeking something. Again we must be careful not to label such behaviour as 'wandering'. There are many reasons for walking about. The person, as Graham Stokes says, can be 'pottering with purpose, or searching for their past – going to work, seeking children, seeking security'
- finding comfort. An example of this might be the person who likes to carry objects around with them. This might be anything from a cushion, to a spoon or a soft toy. Holding something meaningful can give the person a sense of purpose as well as comfort and unless it is risky, they should not be discouraged.

In his book 'Challenging Behaviour in Dementia' (2000), Graham Stokes talks about the reasons for apparently 'difficult' behaviour. For example, people who are incontinent or use an inappropriate receptacle may need more support being helped to the toilet and we may need to work harder to look at the behaviour associated with needing to go to the toilet. This might include 'fiddling' with clothing, restlessness, and 'seeking behaviour'.

What do we mean by aggression? We must take care when we describe a person as aggressive. It is more helpful to describe the actual behaviour rather than use subjective language. People may hit, slap, nip, bite and so on.

Remember, 'aggression' may be a defensive reaction. Think about a time when you have had to assist a colleague to support a person with dementia because of some agitated behaviour. How many people went to help? Did you invade the person's personal space? Did you use raised voices? It is very easy to escalate a situation and so we must be mindful of the impact we have on the person with dementia. How would you feel if several people rushed towards you, all talking at once? The person with dementia may not understand what the problem is and only see this as an act of provocation.

Behaviour that is causing concern should be assessed by a mental health professional, but there are things you can do to help, like using an 'ABC' chart.

A = Antecedent. What was happening before the incident/behaviour? What was the person doing, who was with them, what was the environment like, for example was it noisy?

B = Behaviour. Describe the actual behaviour, the length and intensity of the episode. Who else was involved? What, if any, intervention helped?

C = Consequences. What was the result of the behaviour for the person and the other people involved?

Use of ABC charts can help us to look at patterns of behaviour and understand the triggers for that behaviour. Once we have done that we can establish some protective measures and take action to prevent the triggers occurring.

Person centred care planning can also help in identifying the reasons for behaviour and how to support the person.

Case Study

 2.2 **Mr Jones**

Mr Jones is a retired farmer. He likes his own company and spends a lot of time walking about his care home, 'checking his animals'. For several days he has been very upset and in particular has pushed several people out of the way. Two new residents have recently been admitted and Mr Jones has also been coughing a lot.

Thinking about behaviour, other contributory factors and ABC charts, how could you understand what could be happening here?

2.3 **Analyse ways of responding to the behaviour of an individual with dementia, taking into account the abilities and needs of the individual, carers and others**

Tom Kitwood talks about 'Malignant Social Psychology' and 'Positive Person Work'. Responding to the behaviour of a person with dementia depends on the attitudes and values of carers and others. Malignant Social Psychology has 17 elements, including:

- **Intimidation** – making the person frightened by using threats. This type of behaviour might occur when the carer or other person is trying to make the person with dementia do something.

- **Withholding** – refusing to give asked for attention. This can happen when the person with dementia is asking for help repeatedly, or attaches themselves to a carer and is unable to disengage so the carer ignores them.

- **Infantilisation** – treating the person with dementia as a child. It is not uncommon to hear carers and others talk about people with dementia being 'like children' or patronising the person with demeaning language, 'that's a good girl' spoken to a person with dementia who succeeded in eating independently, is an example.

- **Invalidation** – when we fail to recognise the reality of a person with dementia. We might feel uncomfortable or awkward entering another reality and therefore refuse to participate in an interaction with the person.

- **Disempowerment** – when the person with dementia is not allowed to use the abilities they do have. It is difficult sometimes for carers and others to 'let go' because they are afraid the person will come to harm. Such caring behaviour can mean that carers and others become 'risk averse' and do not support the strengths of the person with dementia.

If people work together as a team or carers are supporting a family member, these attitudes can 'spread', particularly if the carers and others have not received training or support in the needs of the person with dementia. They may take their lead from each other and then this 'malignant' cycle must be broken.

There is an alternative way of interacting, working in a positive person centred way. Some of these ways of interacting are:

- **Belonging** – this involves providing a sense of acceptance regardless of the person's abilities. Carers and family members and others are able to accept the person as they are, making them feel valued and respected.
- **Including** – when carers and others are able to encourage the person to feel included in the life of the care home, or their social network or family.
- **Empowerment** – this means that carers and others have an understanding of the needs of the person and respect their dignity as an adult, and in doing so let go of control and support them in making the most of their skills and abilities.
- **Validation** – by doing this carers and others feel comfortable entering into the reality of the person and understand that 'feelings matter most'.
- **Enabling** – carers and others are able to recognise and encourage the person's ability to get involved in an activity within their own capacity.

Time to reflect

(2.3) Responding to individuals with dementia

Christine Bryden says about people with dementia 'As we become more emotional and less cognitive, it's the way you talk to us, not what you say that we will remember. We know the feeling, but don't know the plot. Your smile, your laugh and your touch are what we will connect with ... we're still here, in emotion and spirit, if only you could find us'.

Christine Bryden, *Dancing with Dementia*, (2005) p. 138.

What is Christine's message to carers, families and others? How is she suggesting we respond to people with dementia?

LO3 Be able to communicate positively with an individual who has dementia by valuing their individuality

 Show how the communication style, abilities and needs of an individual with dementia can be used to develop their care plan

When we use care plans in a person centred way, they will help us to support the person in significant areas of their life. Care planning is based on assessments of the person. These assessments should not just include outcomes related to the support the person may need with activities of daily living but should include how they communicate, their skills and needs in terms of communication and interaction.

Research and investigate

(3.1) Care planning

Look at some care plans in the area you work. How well do they reflect the communication strengths, needs and preferences of the people you support? How could you improve the care plan?

Care plans are not fixed in time. They should be adapted to reflect changes in the person's needs and abilities. It is also important to use the care plan as a 'living' piece of information rather than a tick box exercise. Use the care plan to guide you when thinking about how to interact effectively and ensure that new staff are made familiar with the plan. Care plans can also be used in conjunction with other portrayals of the person's strengths and needs. They should be used in conjunction with the personal profile and life story. Each piece of information helps to build this holistic approach to person centred care.

3.2 **Demonstrate how the individual's preferred method/s of interacting can be used to reinforce their identity and uniqueness**

We are all unique. This does not change in the person with dementia – remember, 'person first'. Although the experience of dementia will affect and change methods of interaction, it will not stop it. We must therefore 'tap in' to the person's preferred ways of interacting.

The way we respond to each other and the world around us is part of our identity.

Evidence activity

3.2 Preferred methods of interaction

Think about the staff you work with. When you work or socialise in a group there will be differences in people's preferred methods of interaction. For example, some people will be tactile – that is, happy to exchange a kiss or handshake. Others may be reluctant to speak but will indicate their interest by joining in laughter or holding eye contact. Now think about some of the people you support. What have you noticed about their unique methods of interaction?

Key terms

Tactile means the use of touch to communicate.

We also interact with each other in the context of our social environment. We use particular circumstances as opportunities to interact with individuals or groups. These might be casual, informal events like meeting for coffee, to structured situations like clubs and evening classes. It is vital that we have knowledge of the person with dementia's interests and hobbies. This, as we know, is part of life story work. It may not always be practical or appropriate because of risk issues to accommodate all these interests, but they do reinforce the individual's personhood

or uniqueness and therefore we must enable them to have as many opportunities as possible to continue with their preferred forms of social interaction.

LO4 Be able to use positive interaction approaches with individuals with dementia

4.1 **Explain the differences between a reality orientation approach to interactions and a validation approach**

Reality orientation (RO) describes a method of interaction where we try to place the person in the present, reminding them of the day, place, time and situation they are in. This is one of the first positive interventions that were used with people with dementia. It was developed in the 1950s and introduced to the support of people with dementia in the late 1950s.

The main principle of RO is a positive belief that people with dementia have the right to be brought back to a 'normal' way of life. When we use the RO approach we are encouraging the person to live more in the here and now. In order to do this we need to use prompts, cues and signals. The environment should reflect the current time so it is important to use 'natural' devices like newspapers and diaries, and to consistently refer to current activities and events. For example, when a care worker is supporting a person with dementia to get up in the morning, they will talk about the day of the week, the time of day and give the person a point of reference by indicating that breakfast is the next meal. It is also common practice to use 'RO boards' which show the date, season, names of staff, mealtimes and so on.

The validation approach (VA) was developed by Naomi Feil in the early 1980s. It uses a non-judgemental acceptance and empathy to show the individual that their expressed feelings are valid. This approach focuses on the feelings rather than the content of speech. David Sheard also encourages this method, saying that 'feelings matter most'. Using VA means that we do not scrutinise the meaning of the words, but rather look for the emotional message behind the words, or the place the person may feel themselves to be in. For example, the person constantly seeking 'mother' will not merely be indicating that they have forgotten that their mother has died, they are actually seeking what mother represents – comfort and security.

Reflect on these two forms of interaction

What do you think are the benefits? Are there any disadvantages?

 Demonstrate a positive interaction with an individual who has dementia

Think about the activities you enjoy and the things that comfort you. Is this happening for the person with dementia? If not, how can you improve their situation? Take another look at their care plan and their life story and personal profile. Talk to their family and friends. Can they support the person in an interaction, or give you some ideas about how you can enable the person to interact more positively?

Think about how you are communicating with the person during an interaction. Are you using a model of positive personhood, or is it a case of malignant psychology?

In order to demonstrate a positive interaction with the person you must demonstrate:

- active listening
- responding to the emotions behind the words
- entering the person's reality
- looking for triggers and de-escalating potentially challenging situations
- using different forms of communication, remembering that speaking is only a small part of effective communication
- understanding how the person uses their body language to communicate.

Research and investigate

'The Bridge'

Naomi Feil talks to Gladys Wilson. Use a search engine to find this interaction, from 'The Bridge'. Gladys has advanced dementia and Naomi is able to communicate in an empathetic way which enables Gladys to interact in a meaningful and very moving way.

 Demonstrate how to use aspects of the physical environment to enable positive interactions with individuals with dementia

We all respond to our physical environment, whether that is the comfort of home, or the fun of the seaside, or the peace of a cathedral. Our personhood and spirituality is enriched by the physical environment.

The physical environment must hold significance and meaning for the person with dementia. Remember the social model of disability and how a confusing or bland environment can prevent the person relating to their surroundings.

The senses can be stimulated by the environment. The life of the person with dementia can be enriched by:

- sensory gardens
- the use of music. It is helpful to use different types of music to indicate times of the day – for example, quiet soothing music at night and more lively music during the day. Play music that is age appropriate and that relates to the time of the year when possible.
- colour coded doors, door furniture, toilet seats and so on. Use good signage that does not rely just on words, but symbols and pictures that are meaningful.
- 'breaking up' bland corridors with interesting themed features. Encourage people to personalise their bedroom doors and use ideas to enable people to more easily recognise their environment. For example, in a care home, you might give each corridor a street name and decorate the walls accordingly.
- a warm, interesting environment which will give a positive message. Individualised rooms help the person maintain their sense of identity and personhood. Life stories and personal profiles will help to create an environment that is meaningful.

Dos and don'ts

Write a short 'dos and don'ts' list for carers to give them some ideas about how to adapt the physical environment for the person with dementia. You could also use magazine cuttings, fabric swatches and so on to illustrate your work.

4.4 Demonstrate how to use aspects of the social environment to enable positive interactions with individuals with dementia

The physical environment describes the space in which we live and the social environment is the network of friends, family and wider society to which we belong. Our social environment is complex because we develop different relationships, depending on our circumstances. For example, think about the different relationships you have with your manager and your mother, or your friends or the person who serves you in a shop. This means we have a rich variety of experiences and these can be used to good effect for the person with dementia.

Social inclusion is vital – that is, being an active part of a social network and society. It is important for the person to interact with the person in the shop as well as their family, for example. All positive relationships should be encouraged, and by doing so, social skills are maintained for longer. Continuing the social routine – going to the hairdressers, meeting friends for coffee or going to the pub are all examples of maintaining social inclusion.

Family and friends can help by talking about past events and happy memories. This is important for the person's sense of 'self' because their family and friends share a personal, cultural and historical perspective.

Engagement in familiar activities like going to church or a mosque as part of the person's spirituality, or going to bingo or for walks in the country enrich and fulfil longstanding personal needs.

Meaningful occupations like films, music, carpet games, singing for the brain, circle dancing and themed parties are all positive ways of interaction and stimulation.

4.5 Demonstrate how reminiscence techniques can be used to facilitate a positive interaction with the individual with dementia

We have learnt that there are several methods of supporting the person with dementia when communicating. It is important that you modify your approach, depending on the person themselves, the stage they are in their dementia and the emotions they are feeling. Reminiscence techniques are very helpful for people who find great difficulty relating to a current reality and whose memories are more long term.

We have learnt that people's reality may be focused on a significant time in their life, possibly when they were much younger. Reminiscence techniques based on recalling past events and achievements support the person in their reality. They are a way of relating to the person in a meaningful way by sharing their memories and 'drawing out' their recollections.

Reminiscence can be done in a general or more specific way. Watching old films, for example, can stimulate memories and conversations, and looking at family photographs will generate a more personal response. Artefacts like household objects, clothes, postcards and so on can be used in the immediate environment to bring back memories and give focus to discussion.

It is important to be age appropriate. Consider the generation and age of the person you are communicating and interacting with. Do not assume their memories are based on the 'war years'. It is likely that they belong to the next generation now. Think about their current age and 'count back' to when they were busy with family life. This is where most vivid memories may lie, and this might be in the 1950s and 1960s.

▌Research and investigate

4.4 Using the social environment

Look at the care plans for the people you support. How much do they take into account the use of the social environment? How could you maintain social inclusion for the people you support, using a person centred approach?

Evidence activity

4.5 Using reminiscence techniques

Compile a 'memory or reminiscence' resource for the people you support. Collect items from everyday life, books, films, postcards, recipes and so on. You could design a poster asking for donations from families or colleagues. Consider how you might use the resource, both on a one-to-one basis or in a group (but avoid the 'classroom' approach!).

Assessment Summary DEM 312

Reading this unit and completing the activities will have provided you with knowledge, understanding and skills required to understand and enable interaction and communication with individuals who have dementia.

To achieve the unit, your assessor will require you to:

Learning Outcomes	Assessment Criteria
1 Understand the factors that can affect communication and interaction with individuals who have dementia	**1.1** Explain how different forms of dementia may affect the way an individual communicates See evidence activity 1.1, page 85
	1.2 Explain how physical and mental health factors may need to be considered when communicating with an individual who has dementia See case study 1.2, page 85
	1.3 Describe how to support different communication abilities and needs of an individual with dementia who has a sensory impairment See time to reflect 1.3, page 86
	1.4 Describe the impact the behaviour of carers and others may have on an individual with dementia See evidence activity 1.4, page 87
2 Be able to communicate with an individual with dementia using a range of verbal and non-verbal techniques	**2.1** Demonstrate how to use different communication techniques with an individual who has dementia See evidence activity 2.1, page 88
	2.2 Show how observation of behaviour is an effective tool in interpreting needs of an individual with dementia See case study 2.2, page 89
	2.3 Analyse ways of responding to the behaviour of an individual with dementia, taking account of the abilities and needs of the individual, carers and others See time to reflect 2.3, page 90

Learning Outcomes	Assessment Criteria
3 Be able to communicate positively with an individual who has dementia by valuing their individuality	Show how the communication style, abilities and needs of an individual with dementia can be used to develop their care plan See research and investigate 3.1, page 90
	Demonstrate how the individual's preferred method/s of interacting can be used to reinforce their identity and uniqueness See evidence activity 3.2, page 91
4 Be able to use positive interaction approaches with individuals with dementia	Explain the differences between a reality orientation approach to interactions and a validation approach See evidence activity 4.1, page 92
	Demonstrate a positive interaction with an individual who has dementia See research and investigate 4.2, page 92
	Demonstrate how to use aspects of the physical environment to enable positive interactions with individuals with dementia See evidence activity 4.3, page 92
	Demonstrate how to use aspects of the social environment to enable positive interactions with individuals with dementia See research and investigate activity 4.4, page 93
	Demonstrate how reminiscence techniques can be used to facilitate a positive interaction with the individual with dementia See evidence activity 4.5, page 93

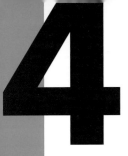

Equality, Diversity and Inclusion in Dementia Care
DEM 207 Understand equality, diversity and inclusion in dementia care

What are you finding out?

Diversity is defined as being when many numerous types of things or people are part of something. For individuals with dementia in a health and social care setting it is important for diversity to be prominent and respected. Recognising diversity allows for a more inclusive approach to care and support and ensures the effective delivery of person centred care.

This unit is aimed at those who provide care or support to individuals with dementia in a wide range of settings. The unit introduces the concepts of equality, diversity and inclusion that are fundamental to person centred care practice.

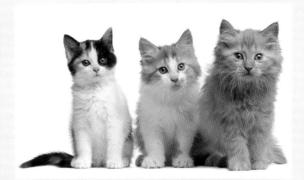

Figure 4.1 We can see diversity all around us. We must recognise that we are unique individuals but that we all share personhood whatever our race, disability or gender.

Reading this unit and completing the activities will allow you to:

• Understand and appreciate the importance of diversity of individuals with dementia

• Understand the importance of person centred approaches in the care and support of individuals with dementia

• Understand ways of working with a range of individuals who have dementia to ensure diverse needs are met

LO1 Understand and appreciate the importance of diversity of individuals with dementia

In this section we will consider the importance of diversity, equality and inclusion in dementia care and support. It is crucial to understand and appreciate the importance of diversity due to the unique experience of dementia and the ways in which quality of life can be improved. Understanding issues of diversity recognises the person as well as the dementia.

1.1 Explain the importance of recognising that individuals with dementia have unique needs and preferences

Each and every person was born into different families, different circumstances, made different choices and had different life experiences. Difference is what makes each and every one of us unique. Tom Kitwood says: 'when you have met one person with dementia you have met just one person with dementia'. Not everyone with dementia is the same. As we will discuss throughout this chapter, equality, diversity and inclusion means understanding that all people are individuals who have unique needs and preferences. This includes taking people's tastes, skills, preferences, habits and behaviours and so on into consideration. It is important to recognise that not everyone that you will be supporting will like or behave in the same way as someone else. This is because everyone is unique. If everyone was the same then we would behave the same way towards people, expect them to eat the same food, wear the same clothes and have the same religious background.

Every person that we interact with is different.

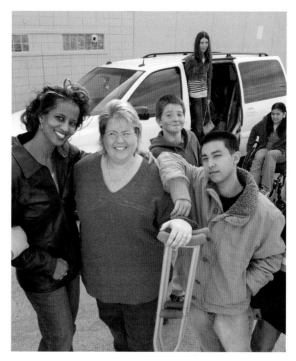

Figure 4.2 Our life experiences shape all of us.

1.2 Describe ways of helping carers and others to understand that an individual with dementia has unique needs and preferences

It is important that as carers we understand why we gather as much information as possible about the people we care for. It is essential that we have insight into the backgrounds of the people that we work with, our families and friends so that we can have meaningful social interactions with the people around us. This also applies to individuals living with dementia. Understanding unique needs and preferences allows us to provide a good and positive way of working and caring for others but also generates a genuine interest in another person's life. This knowledge can be useful when promoting positive interactions but also when trying to understand another person's behaviour. If someone is upset because their unique needs are not being met then they may communicate this through behaviour.

Evidence activity

1.2 Understanding unique needs and preferences

This activity will encourage you to consider ways of helping carers and others to understand that an individual with dementia has unique needs and preferences.

1. Ask a carer about what their favourite way to relax after a long day is.

2. Then ask them how they might feel if for whatever reason they could not do the things they like to do to relax.

3. Identify their unique needs and preferences.

1.3 Explain how values, beliefs and misunderstandings about dementia can affect attitudes towards individuals

There are still a lot of myths and misunderstandings around dementia. This could be because dementia tends to affect old people, although we have discussed how dementia can affect younger people too. Old people tend to be stigmatised due to ageism.

Key terms

Discrimination is unfair treatment of a person, based on prejudice.

Stigma is prejudice based upon stereotyped beliefs and values about others.

Prejudice is a negative judgement or opinion formed in advance or without knowledge of the facts.

Ageism is discrimination against people on the grounds of age; in this case specifically, discrimination against the elderly.

Dementia is also associated with or linked to mental health. Mental health is also a term that some people find threatening. Often it is deemed weird or scary for some people to think about mental health because it is still viewed in a negative way. The way we view our world is influenced by the way we value things and people and the relationships that exist between them. We learn our values and beliefs by our own life experiences and by what we learn from others. The ways in which we form our beliefs structure our own preconceptions. This is called socialisation. We are socialised by the groups and individuals we socialise with who may have preconceived ideas about what dementia means and the individuals who develop it.

Key terms

Socialisation is the process of modifying behaviours, beliefs and values from infancy throughout the life course.

Therefore there will be different values and belief systems of dementia that can lead to misunderstandings. The myths around dementia could be, s/he is behaving like that because s/he is stubborn, mischievous or naughty. Dementia only happens to old people. Or people get better from dementia. All of these different beliefs and values affect attitudes.

Key terms

Attitude is the total sum of beliefs and values that lead to a way of behaving towards something or someone.

If values and beliefs about dementia are lacking in understanding then this can lead to unfair attitudes. These types of attitudes can be negative towards individuals with dementia and lead to them being treated in ways that they really do not deserve. This is because they have been misunderstood.

Case Study

1.3 Tomas

A new member of staff is talking in the staff room about an individual with dementia. The individual is called Tomas and likes to walk around the care home and tidy as he goes. In particular he takes great care and

continued ...

consideration in straightening the pictures in the corridors. He is a Polish gentleman and was a housekeeper for a wealthy family. The member of staff says that he should not be allowed to walk around because he could be dangerous. The member of staff is concerned that because he doesn't speak English he will not understand prompts for meals.

Tomas is still physically well and still has the capacity to make a sandwich and he also enjoys socialising with people he meets around the home.

1) Describe the new member of staff's attitude.

2) What values, beliefs and misunderstandings about dementia does the new member of staff have?

3) How could these affect Tomas
   - physically
   - socially?

LO2 Understand the importance of person centred approaches in the care and support of individuals with dementia

A person centred approach to care and support is fundamental to all aspects of health and social care. For people with dementia it is particularly important that we ensure that their individuality, needs, wishes and wellbeing are at the centre of all we do to support them. Put simply, we must always see the person first and not the dementia. No two people with dementia are the same.

 Describe how an individual may feel valued, included and able to engage in daily life

We all need to feel valued and included and able to engage or fit into daily life. Our routines are important to us because we have roles in life that means that we do things for ourselves and others that are meaningful. These things make us feel valued because we are needed and our actions have an important effect on others and the way we feel about our self. The ways in which an individual with dementia may feel valued, included and able to engage in daily life can have an effect on their mental wellbeing and physical health. The ways in which individuals can engage in daily life will depend on lots of different factors and may fluctuate or change from one day to the next. One day may be better than another. Every individual has different interests, roles and talents. In the same vein, there are activities and pastimes that some people do not like. We have different likes and dislikes because everyone is unique. It is important to understand what roles individuals like to take, their pastimes and interests to assist them in participating in daily life. For example, one person may like setting the table whilst another may like gardening or tidying up. Understanding what makes people tick and helping them to achieve and realise those interests can help them feel included and valued in daily life.

Case Study

(2.1) **Tomas**

Tomas is a Polish gentleman who used to be a housekeeper for a wealthy family. He is still physically well and enjoys walking around the home tidying as he goes and chatting to people he meets along the way. The housekeeper works in the laundry on Thursdays and she puts new cushion covers on all the chairs and pairs socks. There are two other people who work in the laundry who also work on activities. They find that Tomas really enjoys coming along and helping in the laundry and have found that his arthritic fingers have benefitted from the movement of pairing socks. His coordination is good and he also tells stories of his childhood in Poland and his experience of working as a housekeeper.

1) In what ways does Tomas feel valued?

2) In what ways does Tomas feel included?

3) In what ways does Tomas feel able to engage in daily life
   - physically
   - socially?

2.2 Describe how individuals with dementia may feel excluded

We have all felt excluded at some point in our lives. To be excluded means that we do not get the opportunity to or cannot participate in something that we could or might want to. This could be for a variety of reasons. Perhaps we could not play with the older children when we were little because it was too dangerous or we did not know how to play the game. Perhaps there was an older child or sibling that would not let us. As we discussed in Chapter 1 individuals with dementia still have the right to participate in activities but because of discrimination, oversight or a lack of or diminishing skill set may not feel able to. A single invitation to be part of something that is happening or being included in a conversation can prevent someone feeling excluded or left out. Individuals with dementia can also feel excluded or left out of decision-making processes so it is important to include them at meetings or events when consultations may take place.

Case Study

2.2 Tomas

Tomas has just been told by the new member of staff that he must sit in the living room. The television is on very loud with Jeremy Kyle blaring across the room. The room is set out with chairs around the outside of the room and the person he is sitting next to is asleep. Tomas has waited for a member of staff so that he can ask if he should go and help in the laundry. He is anxious because he should be working. Because the television is so loud and he doesn't understand the language he becomes more upset and shouts. The new member of staff says to her colleague that this confirms what she had thought.

In what ways is Tomas being excluded?

Physically?

1)

2)

3)

Socially?

1)

2)

3)

 2.3 Explain the importance of including the individual in all aspects of their care

It is important to include individuals with dementia in all aspects of their care so that their needs and wishes can be met. It is also important to make sure that individuals are consulted on a regular basis so that levels of care and support can be evaluated. This type of inclusion means that any changes can be addressed and care plans modified. A care plan should be specific and tailored to the individual with dementia and their carer. It should be written in a way that reflects an understanding of their perspective and life experiences. By including the person as much as possible, the process will be more helpful and they are more likely to 'own' the care plan. They may be able to write their own plan with you so that it is an individualised care plan that reflects individual needs with the capacity to be responsive to change.

Case Study

2.3 Tomas

This week Tomas's care plan is due to be updated and you are the support worker who will be responsible for discussing Tomas's needs.

1) Who will you speak to first?

2) Why will you speak to this person?

3) Are there any recent developments that you think should be included?

LO3 Understand ways of working with a range of individuals who have dementia to ensure diverse needs are met

Throughout this chapter we have discussed how a range of individuals can develop dementia and emphasised that each individual is unique. When working with a range of individuals a diverse set of needs should be considered to provide care and support that is person centred.

3.1 Describe how the experience of an older individual with dementia may be different from the experience of a younger individual with dementia

Older people are generally more accepting of care, and service provision could be more likely orientated towards the issues that an older person with dementia may encounter. Older people may be of pensionable age and have no work commitments. Younger people with dementia are classified as being under 65 years old. It is estimated that there are around 16,000 to 25,000 younger people with dementia.

Physically, older people will experience aspects of the natural ageing process such as visual impairment, hearing impairment, limited mobility, or dexterity and are perhaps a little more accepting of the changes that they are experiencing physically.

Socially, older people may not experience the types of social networks that a younger person may have. Families and friends may also be elderly and have conditions and illness that impair them. Older people tend to be socially excluded and do not participate in everyday outings like younger people may do.

3.2 Describe what steps might be taken to gain knowledge and understanding of the needs and preferences of individuals with dementia from different ethnic origins

Individuals with dementia come from a variety of backgrounds. These include different ethnic backgrounds. Individuals from different ethnic backgrounds have varying needs and preferences such as food, religion, language, dress, customs and heritage. Therefore it is important that these diverse needs are explored and understood. There are a number of steps that can be taken to understand the needs and preferences of individuals from different ethnic backgrounds.

- **Life story work** – understanding the life story of an individual can give you immediate access to information that can be used to ensure needs are met. Life story work can also provide clues and knowledge that can be used for further exploration.

- **Family and friends** – talking with the family and friends of individuals with dementia from ethnic backgrounds can assist you in compiling information that assists your understanding of their needs and preferences as a family unit and what is important to them.

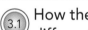
Evidence activity

3.1 How the experience of an older individual with dementia may be different from the experience of a younger individual with dementia

In the table below list similarities and differences between an older and younger person's experience of dementia.

Older person with dementia	Younger person with dementia	Similarities	Differences

- **Independent research** – you could also carry out some research of your own into cultures and ethnic backgrounds.

Evidence activity

 3.2 Steps that might be taken to gain knowledge and understanding of the needs and preferences of individuals with dementia from different ethnic origins

Abda is a Hungarian lady who does not speak English. She has one sister and a friend who are both elderly. What steps could you take to get to know more about Hungarian culture and Abda's personal experiences?

 3.3 Describe what knowledge and understanding would be required to work in a person centred way with an individual with a learning disability and dementia

Individuals with a learning disability can present behaviours that challenge and this is compounded when they develop dementia. It is crucial that staff and service providers are aware of specific knowledge and issues concerning the individuals that they care for and support so that a person centred approach can be facilitated.

An individual with a learning disability may have difficulties with:

- living skills
- health problems – which can mimic dementia symptoms

- communication
- unreliable history
- generic assessments
- misdiagnosis.

The difficulties cited above are similar to some of those that are experienced with dementia. Therefore it is vital that these are closely monitored so that changes and/or fluctuation in capabilities can be noted to maintain skills sets, independence and dignity.

Evidence activity

3.3 What knowledge and understanding would be required to work in a person centred way with an individual with a learning disability and dementia?

To take into account the individual's current and past interests, preferences and needs and work in a person centred way:

- Create a box of memories or life story book.
- Use visual or pictorial cues to orientate them.

Think about:

- What alternative ways of communicating could be used?
- How are their eating and drinking skills?
- What are their favourite foods?
- What are their specific interests and preferences?

What other knowledge and understanding do you think may be useful?

Assessment Summary DEM 207

Your reading of this unit and completion of the activities will have prepared you to care for or give support to individuals with dementia in a wide range of settings. The unit introduces the concepts of equality, diversity and inclusion that are fundamental to person centred care practice.

To achieve the unit, your assessor will require you to:

Learning Outcomes	Assessment Criteria
1 Understand and appreciate the importance of diversity of individuals with dementia	**1.1** Explain the importance of recognising that individuals with dementia have unique needs and preferences **See evidence activity 1.1, page 97**
	1.2 Describe ways of helping carers and others to understand that an individual with dementia has unique needs and preference **See evidence activity 1.2, page 98**
	1.3 Explain how values, beliefs and misunderstandings about dementia can affect attitudes towards individual **See case study 1.3, page 98**
2 Understand the importance of person centred approaches in the care and support of individuals with dementia	**2.1** Describe how an individual may feel valued, included and able to engage in daily life **See case study 2.1, page 99**
	2.2 Describe how individuals with dementia may feel excluded **See case study 2.2, page 100**
	2.3 Explain the importance of including the individual in all aspects of their care **See case study 2.3, page 100**
3 Understand ways of working with a range of individuals who have dementia to ensure diverse needs are met	**3.1** Describe how the experience of an older individual with dementia may be different from the experience of a younger individual with dementia **See evidence activity 3.1, page 101**
	3.2 Describe what steps might be taken to gain knowledge and understanding of the needs and preferences of individuals with dementia from different ethnic origins **See evidence activity 3.2, page 102**
	3.3 Describe what knowledge and understanding would be required to work in a person centred way with an individual with a learning disability and dementia **See evidence activity 3.3, page 102**

DEM 209 Equality, diversity and inclusion in dementia care practice

What are you finding out?

In this unit we will look at how we must, in person centred care practice, take into account the uniqueness of each person by understanding the importance of equality, diversity and inclusion. In health and social care we inevitably work with a wide range of people of different ages, cultures, social and religious backgrounds and with different needs and expectations. It is our responsibility to see each person as an individual in the context of their personal history – what makes them unique. We must remember, 'person' first, 'dementia' second.

Reading the unit and completing the activities will allow you to:

- Understand the importance of equality, diversity and inclusion when working with individuals with dementia

- Be able to apply a person centred approach in the care and support of individuals with dementia

- Be able to work with a range of individuals who have dementia to ensure diverse needs are met

LO1 Understand the importance of equality, diversity and inclusion when working with individuals with dementia

 Explain what is meant by:

- Diversity
- Equality
- Inclusion

These three terms describe some of the fundamental principles of delivering health and social care. They are also key to how our society treats its citizens, and therefore are supported by legislation.

▌Research and investigate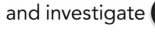

1.1 Legislation

Use a search engine or check other sections in this unit to find out more about the different laws supporting diversity, equality and inclusion.

- **Diversity** describes the broad spectrum of people in any one society. People come from a variety of backgrounds; have different life experiences, views, beliefs and tastes. People with dementia are no different and before we consider how we support the person with dementia, we should start by understanding the unique needs and preferences which have been influenced by their own life history.

- **Equality** means ensuring that all individuals (irrespective of their age, sexuality, race, ethnic background or disability) have the opportunity to live the way they choose, according to their values and beliefs. Equality does not mean treating everyone the same but is about ensuring that people are treated fairly and equitably according to their needs.

- **Inclusion** means being able to participate in mainstream activity. This includes having the right to be included and acknowledged in all aspects of society.

▌Time to reflect

1.1 Inclusion

Reflect on a situation when you felt 'left out' or excluded from a group of people or a situation. How did it make you feel? Why do you think that some people are excluded from the mainstream? This happens to people with dementia, can you think of other groups of people who are excluded from some aspects of society?

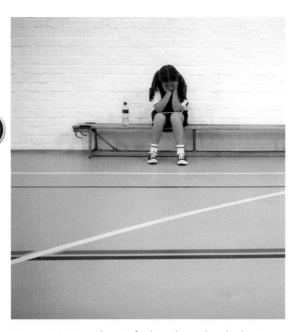

Figure 4.3 How does it feel to always be the last to be picked for the team. Would it make you feel discriminated against?

1.2 Explain why an individual with dementia has unique needs and preferences

If we accept that we are all unique then inevitably we are also accepting that each person with dementia is different with their own needs and preferences. They may have a similar condition, but as we have already learnt in Chapter 1, dementia affects each person in a different way. This is how we put person centred care into action. It recognises that by **not** meeting the person's unique needs and preferences we will ignore their personhood and probably cause some of the 'difficult' behaviour that is often mistakenly but automatically associated with dementia.

Tom Kitwood describes the main psychological needs of a person with dementia as having five overlapping needs with love at the centre (Figure 4.4).

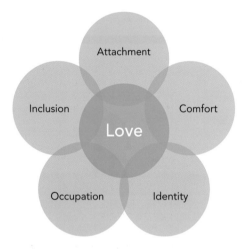

Figure 4.4 The main psychological needs of a person with dementia.
Tom Kitwood *Dementia Reconsidered* 1997.

If we look at these needs we can see that in fact they can relate to all of us because they are part of our personhood.

As well as inclusion, Tom Kitwood suggests a person with dementia needs to feel they are occupied in a purposeful way (consider how you feel when you are bored or unable to join in an activity). Our occupation, family, history and culture give us a sense of identity. We have feelings of comfort and attachment when we are included and valued.

If we recognise the unique needs and preferences of people with dementia we are:

- looking beyond the label and seeing the person
- promoting the person's wellbeing
- ensuring they have choices and we respect their privacy and dignity.

Research and investigate

1.2 Promoting needs and preferences

Look at some care plans. How do they reflect the unique needs and preferences of the person? How could you improve the care plan? What other ways could you ensure that all care workers are aware of the unique needs and preferences of the person?

1.3 **Describe how an individual with dementia may feel excluded**

Societies have often excluded people who are different to the main population or who are seen to be a threat of some kind. This has been the case, for example, for people from ethnic minorities, or people with a disability. Older people often feel excluded because society has tended to see them as a burden and in need of support. We rely on stereotypes to support this idea, that is, all people who are older and frail rely on other people, or that all people with dementia are difficult and unable to cope in society.

This is not the case. Tom Kitwood argues that we often exclude people with dementia because we are afraid of them and the illness – but dementia affects us all and it does not distinguish between people. This means that we all face the same reality.

Although the way dementia affects people may differ, the experiences of people in terms of exclusion can often be the same. The early stages of the condition may impact very little on the person and they might continue to attend their social activities, to go shopping, to the library, to clubs and societies and so on. As things progress, so the person with dementia can experience changes, which may be subtle at first – people not talking to them as much at social events because it is not so easy to engage with the person. As the person struggles with their dementia and begins to feel more isolated, friends, neighbours and society in general may also make life more difficult. Some environments are not always suitable for the person, or their friends lack understanding and are unable to communicate with the person so stop trying. Families and friends may feel embarrassed about taking the person with dementia into public places and their social life gradually fades away.

Inevitably, the person with dementia can feel unable to mix with other people. Going to the shops can become daunting and they feel excluded when they try to join in their usual activities. There is then a huge danger of social exclusion and isolation.

We can exclude a person with dementia, not just by removing them from activities but by ignoring them or talking over them. If we criticise or shout at the person this reinforces their feelings of being a 'nuisance' and if we use demeaning language (referring to the person in a way that takes away their personhood) they can feel worthless.

daily life. Consider the activities that you undertake and the choices you make without a second thought. Do you like a shower or bath, do you like to stay up late, wear a certain colour or always drink coffee? Imagine how you would feel if these choices were taken away from you.

Person centred care recognises that despite someone's disability they still have the same rights and choices and that as care workers we must ensure that these are not ignored. Task oriented care ignores personhood and there is little effort made to understand the person's needs and choices. This means that actual needs are often 'unmet' because they have not been acknowledged. If the person with dementia is not included they may become withdrawn or agitated. This can become a 'vicious circle' because it can lead to the person being labelled as difficult because they have dementia and are less and less the centre of their own world. We take over and make decisions for them rather than take the time to actively listen and empathise.

Time to reflect

1.3 Exclusion

Christine Bryden talks about her experience of living with dementia in her book *Dancing with Dementia*.

She says: 'Isolation is a real problem for us. Many of us feel that some people even think dementia is contagious! We don't see many friends any more. It seems as if people treat us differently now because they know we have dementia, and they don't know what to do.'

Think about the ways in which people with dementia and their carers can feel less excluded. What services and support networks are there in your local area that can support people with dementia and their social network?

1.4 Describe why it is important to include an individual with dementia in all aspects of care practice

Imagine how you would feel if you were not consulted about or involved in aspects of your

 Evidence activity

1.4 Inclusive practice

Think about three aspects of care practice with a person with dementia. How could you improve your practice in these areas to ensure you are including the person more? Discuss this with your manager and colleagues. Can you reflect this improved practice in their care plan? Think about how you will communicate with the person and demonstrate how you have included them.

1.5 Explain how values, beliefs and misunderstandings about dementia can affect attitudes towards an individual

- **Values** – consider what is important to you and the kind of values you hold about family, friendship, and the way you treat people. If we do not value the status of a person with dementia and the place they have in society we are undermining their personhood.

- **Beliefs** – what kind of things do you believe to be true and how do these beliefs shape your attitudes and actions? If we believe that all people with dementia are unable to think for themselves or have opinions or feelings, we are excluding them from society.

There are some common misunderstandings about dementia, like 'dementia only occurs in older people', or 'people with dementia are always aggressive and cannot take part in normal activities'.

There is an attitude which says that nothing can be done and it is best to accept that a person with dementia just needs 'looking after'. In this way we begin to 'dehumanise' the person with dementia. We stop seeing them as another human being but rather as someone with a medical condition that defines them. This is how we stigmatise and stereotype people with dementia. They are set apart and treated with prejudice and discrimination.

There is the belief that people with dementia forget everything and so there is no point engaging with them. Again, this is not the case. People with dementia may have difficulty with their memory, but their feelings remain. They may not be able to recall an experience but the emotion is real and can stay with the person.

As care workers it is our responsibility to break down those attitudes and help to correct the misunderstandings.

Research and investigate

 1.5 Values, beliefs and misunderstandings

Look at some recent media coverage of dementia issues. Make a list of the negative language and some of the published misunderstandings that could shape the public perception of dementia

LO2 Be able to apply a person centred approach in the care and support of individuals with dementia

This approach ensures that the diversity of the person is acknowledged, that they are treated with equality and included in their own care and support. We discussed this in greater depth in Chapter 2 'Person Centred Care'.

2.1 Demonstrate how an individual with dementia has been valued, included and able to engage in daily life

By valuing the person for who they are and including them we can ensure that they maintain their **sense of identity** and improve their **self-esteem**. Engaging in daily life includes **social inclusion** as well as personal care. If we support people in more involvement in the outside world they can feel more **accepted and valued**.

We know that dementia affects communication and interaction. If the person with dementia is supported in communication and interaction (See Chapter 3 'Communication') they are more likely to feel confident in maintaining and making new social relationships.

Think back to Tom Kitwood's model of psychological needs which include attachment (belonging) and occupation. We can encourage the person to continue with meaningful occupation. This should be done in the context of their dementia 'journey'. If we expect too much of the person we can demoralise them, but if we expect too little they may feel patronised and undervalued. Meaningful occupation for one person may be the ability to dress independently and to enjoy gardening, for another it may be to sing and enjoy their life story book.

Case Study

2.1 Mr Jones

Mr Jones attends a day centre. He used to be a waiter and is constantly following a care assistant about. She is becoming irritated with him, and feels that he is just pestering her. Using a person centred approach, her colleague talks to Mr Jones and listens to his stories about being a waiter. She decides to take action to improve his situation at the day centre. Using the principles of inclusion and valuing people by engaging them in everyday life, what do you think the new person centred approach would include?)

2.2 Show how an individual's life history and culture has been taken into consideration to meet their needs

Life stories and personal profiles are as important for the person with dementia as care plans. We cannot meet a person's needs in a person centred way unless we understand the context of those needs and the person's preferences and values.

Life history includes details about family and social networks, work and leisure experiences. A person's culture explains their view of life, the values they hold dear and the way in which they go about their daily life.

Learning about life history and a person's culture helps us to:

- respect their values and choices and enable them to maintain their personal identity
- support and maintain relationships with their family and social networks
- communicate in a meaningful way
- strengthen our relationship with the person with dementia.

Evidence activity

2.2 Life histories

Write a list of all your needs, including personal care and social, emotional and spiritual needs. Think about how your personal history and culture has shaped those needs. Now imagine you are a person with dementia. Write a care plan explaining how you would expect these needs to be met.

2.3 Demonstrate how the stage of dementia of an individual has been taken into account when meeting their needs and preferences

Each stage and type of dementia affects the person in a different way and this must be remembered in a person centred care approach. There will be some broad similarities, however, and basic principles to consider.

- Ensure you maintain a person rather than task centred approach.
- Use life stories and personal profiles to support your understanding of the person.
- Include the person as much as possible by adapting your communication skills to empower the person with dementia to contribute to their assessment and care plan.
- Include families, friends and carers in your approach.
- Do not rely on assumptions and stereotypes about people with dementia.
- Remember that whatever stage the person may be in, emotions and feelings remain and any experience will have a negative or positive impact depending on your interaction.
- Tailor activities according to the assessed abilities of the person.
- Play to the strengths of the person.
- Do your homework! Improve your understanding of how the person is affected by their dementia and why they are behaving in a particular way.
- Work as a team. People with dementia respond better to a consistent approach. Share information about the person's changing abilities and needs.
- Reassess the person's abilities and needs regularly as you must be aware of any changes in their communication skills, for example. By reassessing you can ensure that the care plan is tailored to meet their needs.
- Adapt activities and environments to meet changing needs. The person with dementia may no longer be able to read a book as the condition changes but they may enjoy looking at a book with you or being read to, or simply holding a book because it is a familiar object and gives them comfort.
- Be aware of changes in the person's mood. They may become more withdrawn and possibly depressed.
- Be aware of the impact physical ill health and medication can have on the person, particularly as they become frailer or the dementia progresses.
- Never forget the person. They are still there and need you to affirm their individuality.

Case Study

2.3 Mr Jones

Mr Jones is no longer able to go to the day centre as he is now very unsettled and feels that he has to leave all the time. The staff are not able to support him safely. He still wants to help out and needs a new outlet for his energies. The Mental Health Nurse reassesses his abilities and needs. Mr Jones indicates that he is lonely. He has the same needs – to be included and occupied.

Consider the options for Mr Jones. What kind of activities and support might be included in the care plan?

2.4 Demonstrate ways of helping carers and others to understand that an individual with dementia has unique needs and preferences

Before we begin it is important that we have an understanding of **the person** with dementia and the actual experience of **dementia**. We have already thought about the misunderstandings and myths surrounding dementia and how people can be stereotyped when they have a diagnosis.

In order to help carers and others to understand that people with dementia have unique needs and preferences we must support them in their understanding of the condition. Educating carers and other professionals as well as the general public is part of the national campaigns we have seen recently. The public information messages have included:

'I have dementia, but I also have a life.'

and

'Dementia, the more we understand, the more we can help'.

This has been generated by the National Dementia Strategy, 'Living Well with Dementia'.

There are practical things we can do to help carers and other professionals. Good communication and trust is key. We can also:

- share life stories and profiles with other professionals on a 'need to know' basis
- share good practice
- support and offer advice and education to carers

- signpost carers to organisations that can support, like Alzheimer's Society, Age UK, MIND, etc
- work with the person with dementia and their carer as partners. People are more likely to share concerns if they feel they are being treated with respect and listened to.
- ensure you are a positive role model by demonstrating a person centred approach to dementia.

Evidence activity

2.4 Supporting needs and preferences

Describe how you could support a carer and the person with dementia to continue to participate in activities and how you could use life story work in a supportive way.

LO3 Be able to work with a range of individuals who have dementia to ensure diverse needs are met

3.1 Demonstrate how to work in ways that ensure that the needs and preferences of individuals with dementia from a diverse range of backgrounds are met

Life experience shapes our expectations and plans for the future. This equally applies to people from different ethnic backgrounds, people with a learning disability or younger people with dementia. Dementia affects people of all backgrounds and in order to work in ways that meet the needs and preferences of individuals we must first learn as much as possible about them. Life story work is invaluable in helping us do this.

In any aspect of care and support it is crucial to respect the diversity of people and to treat each person as an individual. In dementia care we often have to support the person with dementia in an atmosphere of misunderstanding from others. People with dementia can be excluded socially and we must work in an inclusive way.

A 'collective care' setting can reflect the diversity of the general population and the support offered must be flexible enough to acknowledge that diversity. This response may need to reflect different preferences in diet, values and beliefs and communication.

Evidence activity

 3.1 This activity will enable you to demonstrate your understanding of the importance of meeting diverse needs in different settings.

- Think about your friends and colleagues. In what ways do they demonstrate diversity?
- How do you alter your behaviour or language to accommodate that diversity?
- Think about three people that you have supported. Did you consider their diverse needs and values? How as a staff group did you ensure their needs and preferences were met. How could you improve your approach to working in a way that acknowledges diversity in your practice and care planning?

3.2 Describe how the experience of an older individual with dementia may be different from the experience of a younger individual with dementia

Life experience shapes our expectations and plans for the future. This applies to people from different ethnic backgrounds, people with a learning disability or younger people with dementia.

Inevitably the experience of a younger person with dementia will differ to that of an older person. Dementia, as we know is still associated with the ageing process and it can be a great shock to be diagnosed with dementia when you are still of 'working age'. It is difficult to estimate the number of younger people with dementia in the UK – there are probably 16,000 to 25,000 people.

Younger people with dementia will develop the main types of dementia like Alzheimer's disease, but they also are more likely to have fronto temporal dementia and alcohol related dementia than older people.

Onset of dementia for younger people can affect many aspects of their life:

- **Psychological needs**. Dementia arrives at a time when people are still planning their future. They may still be employed or planning their retirement. Although people may be relieved that they have a diagnosis which explains why they have particular problems, they may also feel afraid of what the future holds and suddenly they cannot plan ahead in the same way. People may feel disempowered and de-skilled, they may lose confidence and depression can closely follow.

Evidence activity

 3.2 Different experiences

Describe how this experience may differ for the older person with dementia.

- **Social issues**. Younger people socialise through work and friends and families. They rely on social skills and the ability to adapt to different situations. A diagnosis of dementia can reduce these social contacts. People may find difficulty in adapting to the changing needs of the person with dementia and if they do not 'fit' the profile of that social world they may find themselves gradually excluded.

- **Financial issues**. The younger person with dementia may still be working and relying on their income to support their family. They may still be paying a mortgage and pension contributions. They may worry how the diagnosis will affect insurance, driving their car and being able to do their job. This can put enormous pressure on the person with dementia and their family, particularly as they fear the loss of income and the status employment gives.

- **Relationships**. The younger person may be married and have dependents. A diagnosis of dementia can change relationships. The partner may struggle with a changing role, particularly if they have to take on the role of carer. It can be very hard for families to see the person with dementia change and become dependent themselves.

Evidence activity

 3.2 Different experiences

Describe how this situation might be different for an older person with dementia and their family.

- **Services.** Until recently, services have been designed more for older people with dementia and there are still traditional models of support like care homes or day care that do not offer facilities and services that cater for the specific needs of younger people. This is beginning to change but it can still be a struggle to find appropriate support at the very time the younger person needs to feel that all is not lost and they can have a positive outlook.

Evidence activity

 Comparing experiences

Draw a table showing on one side the issues for an older person with dementia, and on the other the issues for younger people. Think about:
- occupation
- finances
- relationships
- health
- psychological impact
- types of services.

 Describe how to use a person centred approach with an individual with a learning disability and dementia

We can define a 'learning disability' as 'an impairment of intellectual function, or social function'. This means that the person may have problems with dealing with life skills and intellectual reasoning. People with a learning disability are more likely to develop dementia than the rest of the population.

'Valuing People', the national strategy for learning disability emphasises that people with learning disabilities have the same rights as everyone else. This means that in a person centred care approach to a person with a learning disability who also has dementia we must continue to consider and implement the right to make choices, to support the person to be as independent as possible, and to include the person in their care planning.

Just as people with dementia have been labelled and stigmatised in the past, so have people with a learning disability experienced similar prejudices. We must therefore remember all the principles we have learnt about valuing the rights and choices for people with dementia.

Before working with a person with a learning disability and dementia, first understand their abilities, strengths and skills so you have a 'baseline' to better understand any further impact dementia may be having on their cognitive functioning.

The basic rules of the person centred approach are:
- Learn about the person's personality and their coping skills.
- Learn how they usually communicate and express needs and emotions.
- Find out about any other significant health issues.
- Actively listen to the person and look for non verbal as well as verbal clues to what they are telling you. They may have always used a different method of communication and you need to familiarise yourself with that.
- Ensure communication is two way – explain or show the person.
- Find out about the person's life story, their friends, family and networks will be very important to them and you can enable them to maintain that contact.
- Use a personal profile and respect likes, dislikes, preferences, habits, etc. This will help the person to feel valued as well as maintaining a sense of security.
- It is important to engage the expertise of other people who may understand the person and their needs better than you. 'Co-working' is important and may give continuity for the person if they are already used to another service working with them.

Case Study

Joyce Smith

Joyce Smith is admitted to your care home for a short stay while her family are away. She is very apprehensive and feels that her family have left her. Joyce has Downs syndrome and has been diagnosed with dementia for one year. She is 64 years old. How would you help Joyce to settle in? What might you find out about her before her admission and how would you use this information in a person centred way to support her?

Some helpful references:

Alzheimer's Society (2007) *Out of the Shadows*

Bryden C (2005) *Dancing with Dementia*

Kitwood T (1997) *Dementia Reconsidered, The Person Comes First*

National Dementia Strategy, Department of Health 2009

Assessment Summary DEM 209

Your reading of this unit and completion of the activities will provide you with knowledge, understanding and skills for those who provide care or support to individuals with dementia in a wide range of settings.

The unit introduces the concepts of equality, diversity and inclusion that are fundamental to person centred care practice.

To achieve the unit, your assessor will require you too:

Learning Outcomes	Assessment Criteria
1 Understand the importance of equality, diversity and inclusion when working with individuals with dementia	Explain what is meant by: • diversity • equality • inclusion See research and investigate activity 1.1, page 105
	Explain why an individual with dementia has unique needs and preferences See research and investigate activity 1.2, page 106
	Describe how an individual with dementia may feel excluded See time to reflect activity 1.3, page 107
	Describe why it is important to include an individual with dementia in all aspects of care practice See evidence activity 1.4, page 107
	Explain how values, beliefs and misunderstandings about dementia can affect attitudes towards an individual See research and investigate activity 1.5, page 108
2 Be able to apply a person centred approach in the care and support of individuals with dementia	Demonstrate how an individual with dementia has been valued, included and able to engage in daily life See case study 2.1, page 108
	Show how an individual's life history and culture has been taken into consideration to meet their needs See evidence activity 2.2, page 109
	Demonstrate how the stage of dementia of an individual has been taken into account when meeting their needs and preferences See case study 2.3, page 110

Learning Outcomes	Assessment Criteria
	(2.4) Demonstrate ways of helping carers and others to understand that an individual with dementia has unique needs and preferences See evidence activity 2.4, page 110
3 Be able to work with a range of individuals who have dementia to ensure diverse needs are met	(3.1) Demonstrate how to work in ways that ensure that the needs and preferences of individuals with dementia from a diverse range of backgrounds are met See evidence activity 3.1, page 111
	(3.2) Describe how the experience of an older individual with dementia may be different from the experience of a younger individual with dementia See evidence activities 3.2, page 111
	(3.3) Describe how to use a person centred approach with an individual with a learning disability and dementia See case study 3.3, page 112

DEM 310 Understand the diversity of individuals with dementia and the importance of inclusion

What are you finding out?

In Great Britain over 61.8 million people currently populate the country. This population is projected to pass 70 million by 2029. Great Britain is part of Europe which consists of around 50 independent countries or states. Historically, Europe has welcomed people from countries worldwide and as a result has developed a culture and a legal framework that is open-minded to celebrating and protecting difference. The European Union has developed a legal framework that comprises pieces of legislation. These include the Human Rights Act 1998 and the Equalities Act 2010, and Great Britain has incorporated this framework within its legal system to protect its diverse population, help promote differences and strive for equality. For example, after the Second World War a high number of immigrant workers came from the Caribbean and Asian continent. These people worked and helped to promote recovery in the economy and rebuild Great Britain after the war. Some of these people suffered discrimination and oppression due to their differences and so the law had to protect them. This protection served to preserve their identities and now we see elaborate celebrations such as the Notting Hill Carnival. Similarly, we see celebration of gay identities with events such as Pride, but despite all this hard work we still hear reports of abuse and cruelty. Child neglect, racial abuse, social exclusion of older and disabled people, homophobia and exploitation of immigrant workers are common occurrences. You may have even experienced some of this behaviour yourself.

The reading and activities in this unit will help you to:

• Understand the concept of diversity and its relevance to working with individuals who have dementia

• Understand that each individual's experience of dementia is unique

• Understand the importance of working in a person centred way and how this links to inclusion

LO1 Understand the concept of diversity and its relevance to working with individuals who have dementia

Explain what is meant by the terms:
Diversity

Diversity is defined as being when many numerous types of things or people are part of something. For individuals with dementia in a health and social care setting it is important for diversity to be prominent. This is because of the different age groups, different cultures and different ways of thinking. A helpful way of understanding diversity is to think about the last time you were in the town or city centre. Think about how diverse the people were that you saw: did you see people of different cultures; did you see tall people or small people; did you see any older people or disabled people? Do you know any vegetarian or gay people? The elements that make up diversity are present in many areas of the community. Diversity is all around us on our way to work, when we go shopping on the television. When we go about our daily life we all form part of a diverse society. Indeed the term 'Diversity' is the name of a famous dance group because it reflects diversity through various age groups, different cultures and even height differences. Diversity means that as people come from a variety of backgrounds and have different life experiences, so not everyone's views and tastes will be identical. If we use this model, we can begin to recognise diversity by identifying differences and working with this in our everyday living.

Key terms

Diversity means that as people come from a variety of backgrounds and have different life experiences so not everyone's views, beliefs and tastes will be identical.

In health and social care settings we have many different people with different abilities, sexual orientation, ages, sizes and backgrounds.

The General Medical Council defines diversity as 'the difference in the values, attitudes, cultural perspectives, beliefs, ethnic backgrounds, sexuality, skills, knowledge and life experiences of each individual in any group of people'. This definition refers to differences between people and is used to highlight individual needs. Diversity and the need to observe it effectively is covered by legislation. The Equality Act 2010, Disability Act 1995 and Human Rights Act 1998 are examples of this.

Evidence activity

1.1 Explain types of diversity

This activity will show you how you can recognise diversity.

List the diversities in your workplace within these three areas:

Staff	Residents	Visitors	Explain why they are diverse

Key terms

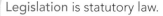

Legislation is statutory law.

The Equality Act 2010 is a framework of legislation that protects the rights of individuals and sets out to advance equal opportunities.

The Human Rights Act 1998 is legislation that sets out and protects individual's fundamental rights.

The General Medical Council is the body that regulates GPs and ensures good medical practice.

Anti-discriminatory practice

Anti-discriminatory practice is about facilitating and promoting equal opportunities by treating everyone equally and in the same way regardless of background. Anti-discriminatory practice can be seen to be applied within the workplace with the integration of particular policies and legislation such as the Equalities Act 2010. In the context of older people an example to demonstrate this philosophy would be to assume that older individuals have the right to have a sex life regardless of age even though they may not be able to perform some everyday tasks like cooking. Another example would be to think about how individuals who use wheelchairs may have limited access to places in comparison to people who do not use wheelchairs.

Time to reflect

 1.1 Ensuring access

What changes could be made to buildings to help make them more accessible?

Anti-oppressive practice

Anti-oppressive practice goes beyond anti-discriminatory practice by challenging the power that is often used by groups or individuals to dominate vulnerable groups and force them into inferior positions. Anti-oppressive practice is about being inclusive in how people behave with, around or towards another person or group of people and seeks to find ways of challenging discriminatory attitudes and oppressive behaviours.

Key terms

Anti-oppressive practice means being inclusive in how people behave with, around or towards another person or group of people and seeks to find ways of challenging discriminatory attitudes and oppressive behaviours.

Anti-oppressive and anti-discriminatory practice are used interchangeably to describe the situation where practitioners treat all people equally in their setting and work to policies such as equal opportunities for all people regardless of culture, disability and gender. You must integrate anti-discriminatory practice in your relationships with people by observing policies that promote equality and inclusion. This ensures that all people are included in activities and exercises. For example, if you were creating a menu, then observing that people who celebrate certain religions may not eat particular foods and then offering alternatives provides opportunities so that they may still feel included.

Evidence activity

 1.1 Anti-discriminatory practice

Think about your workplace, what aspects of it do you think are anti-discriminatory?

1.2 ## Explain why it is important to recognise and respect an individual's heritage

In a health or social care setting there will be many individuals who have come from many different backgrounds, who have had many different experiences, lived in a variety of places, been part of different wars, revolutions, travelled to distant places, never travelled at all, or served with the forces, which can all influence the way the way they form their likes and dislikes. An individual's heritage refers to an individual's culture, history and personal experiences and is unique to them. As a support worker it is vital that you recognise and respect an individual's heritage, which can then provide ideas about some of the key areas that can be considered when thinking about a person's quality of life and what makes them feel happy or may make them feel upset. Understanding an individual's heritage considers how past life experiences could cause their prejudices and therefore facilitates a deeper perceptive and sensitive approach to improving an individual's quality of life. It also provides clues into behaviour that is challenging.

Key terms

Heritage This refers to an individual's culture, history and personal experiences and is unique to them.

1.2 Exploring heritage

Speak to someone that you do not know very well about their background. Ask them about their heritage.

- What is their facial expression?
- How does talking to this person about their heritage make them feel?
- How does it make you feel?

Dementia is not a condition that can be readily seen. Dementia is an invisible condition and is often associated with age and is therefore subject to ageist discrimination. Dementia is also linked to mental health where a large amount of stigma still exists. People can be frightened of dementia because of a lack of understanding and awareness of the issues and challenges faced. In turn, dementia tends to reduce people's status and limit individuals' ability to voice their concerns. Therefore individuals with dementia can receive negative responses primarily because of a lack of understanding and awareness of the issues associated with the condition.

Case Study

1.2 Janice

Janice has recently started to become agitated when going to bed. When Janice's support workers go in to check on her through the night shift they often find her under her bed in uncontrollable tears and very frightened. After Janice's support worker had explored her heritage she found that Janice had survived bombing of the Second World War by lying under a table. She used to keep her windows open so that she could shout for help if she needed it. In her care home the windows were always kept shut.

Janice's support worker found this aspect of Janice's heritage out by talking with her family members. Through this activity it also came to light that Janice liked to garden and grow vegetables when she lived in the countryside. Janice now sleeps through the night since she has her window open and is getting exercise and time outdoors tending to space in the garden.

 1.3 Discrimination

Think of examples of where you have felt that you were discriminated against.

1.
2.
3.

How could an individual with dementia be discriminated against?

1.
2.
3.

 1.4 Describe how discrimination and oppressive practice can be challenged

Discriminative and oppressive practice can be dealt with formally and informally. Often it is about changing or influencing the culture of an organisation. There are also legal channels and policies that can be employed and acted upon to challenge discrimination and oppression. The manner in which the matter is dealt with will depend greatly on the type of negative practice and the severity of it. In every workplace there are clear and accessible routes to challenge discrimination and oppression and if you are in any doubt you should speak with your supervisor or line manager. Challenging discrimination and oppression culturally can be achieved with activities such as positive risk taking. Positive risk

1.3 Describe why an individual with dementia may be subjected to discrimination and oppression

taking can be through encouraging individuals with dementia to participate in activities or roles that they may not have done before. Talking about certain practices among your work colleagues highlighting behaviour that is not tolerated can also promote a work culture that does not accept discrimination and oppression.

Evidence activity

 1.4 Challenging discrimination and oppression

Demonstrate what ways discrimination and oppression can be challenged in your workplace.

Formally

1.

2.

3.

Informally

1.

2.

3.

LO2 Understand that each individual's experience of dementia is unique

Tom Kitwood says: 'When you have met one person with dementia you have met just one person with dementia'. Each and every person was born into different families, different circumstances, made different choices and had different life experiences. Difference is what makes each and every one of us unique. Not everyone with dementia experiences the condition in the same way. The way the brain is affected by dementia depends upon the disease or the condition that is causing it. This affects the symptoms and the way that the dementia will affect the individual. The individual may have more than one type of dementia and other disabilities or health conditions that will affect how dementia is experienced. There are other factors which can affect how dementia is experienced such as social, existing and past skill sets, cultural variations and diverse backgrounds that people come from.

 2.1 Explain why it is important to identify an individual's specific and unique needs

Understanding that every individual with dementia is unique is paramount to good health and social care and support. The diverse backgrounds that make up who we are vital in maintaining cultural traditions such as dress, religion, food, music or decorations, which put together form our self identity. The language that we use or words to describe objects, items, people or parts of our bodies are also essential in our understanding of situations or context. In identifying an individual's unique and specific interests we can address and be sensitive to their cultural background. In doing so mental wellbeing, physical health and social interactions can be greatly improved.

Evidence activity

2.1 Identifying the unique

List five things that show you are a unique person.

How could someone who did not know you identify your unique needs?

2.2 Compare the experience of dementia for an individual who has acquired it as an older person with the experience of an individual who has acquired it as a younger person

Older people are generally more accepting of care, and service provision could be more likely to be orientated towards the issues that an older person with dementia may encounter. An older person may be of pensionable age and have no work commitments. Younger people with dementia are classified as being under 65 years old.

Physically, older people will experience aspects of the natural ageing process such as visual impairment or problems with eyesight, hearing impairment, limited mobility or dexterity and perhaps are a little more accepting of the changes that they are experiencing physically.

Socially, older people may not have the types of social networks that a younger person may have. Families and friends may also be elderly and have conditions and illness that impede them. Older people tend to be socially excluded and do not participate in everyday outings like younger people may do.

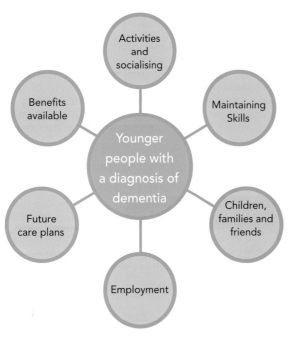

Adapted from: http://www.dementiaweb.org.uk/
younger-people-with-dementia.php

 ## 2.3 Describe how the experience of an individual's dementia may impact on carers

Families and carers of individuals with dementia play an essential role in helping to look after individuals with dementia by assisting with and helping them maintain their independence. Families and carers achieve this through providing ongoing support, care and help with day-to-day tasks for individuals who would otherwise struggle to manage on a day-to-day basis. As we have seen throughout this book, individuals with dementia often present other contributing factors that require specific care such as physical ailments and other symptoms concurrent with the natural ageing process. Physical care requires assistance with bathing, dressing, getting in and out of bed, lifting, toileting, together with the general household activities, which are physically demanding. Fulfilling this role may be compounded and present additional effort especially if the carer is elderly or in poor health themselves. In addition,

Evidence activity

2.3 The impact on carers

A carer walks into your work setting and becomes very upset and fretful. How do you think you could console them? What could be upsetting them?

Evidence activity

2.2 Experiences of dementia

In the table below list similarities and differences between younger and older individuals with dementia.

Older person with dementia	Younger person with dementia	Similarities	Differences

the mental and intellectual challenges families and carers often encounter, such as repetitive questioning, frustrations, orientation, spatial awareness, aphasia and agnosia can be very stressful and mentally arduous. Carers also face a set of behavioural and interpersonal challenges such as constant walking, failing to recognise people, hitting out, forgetting to turn the gas off, sleep disturbance and restlessness.

 2.4 ## Describe how the experience of dementia may be different for individuals

In this section we will describe how the experience of dementia may be different for individuals with learning disabilities, those who come from different ethnic backgrounds and those who are at the end of their life.

Learning disabilities

Individuals with learning disabilities, particularly those with Down's syndrome, are more susceptible to developing dementia in middle age. Due to medical advances people with Down's syndrome are living longer. Individuals with learning disabilities and those with Down's syndrome are also more susceptible to developing visual and hearing impairments. Individuals with Down's syndrome tend to develop dementia earlier at around the age of 55. Individuals with Down's also experience other health problems, which can make dementia difficult to diagnose as the symptoms are somewhat similar.

In terms of care planning, early onset means that individuals with learning disabilities also have a shorter time span for rolling back their history to find out important information that is pertinent to them.

Evidence activity

2.4 Unique experiences of dementia

This activity will help you how you can understand how the experiences of dementia may be different for individuals who have:

- learning disabilities
- are from different ethnic backgrounds
- are at the end of their life.

	Explain why this is important	Who else can help? Team workers Family and friends
What makes the person happy?		
What are the signs of distress or unhappiness?		
Pain management		
Communication		
Important beliefs, cultural, spiritual		

The diagnosis of dementia can be a very negative time for main carers (usually parents). Diagnosis of dementia can bring back the early anxieties often associated with the birth of a child having a learning disability and/or Down's syndrome and what that means to parents. Given the impact of this a carer assessment may be required. Individuals with learning disabilities tend to have a higher reliance on services and so don't tend to have families or support networks.

Different ethnic backgrounds

Ethnic background or ethnicity is where one person identifies with one another through a shared language, faith or religion, specific geographical location and ideology. This unification is often characterised by food, rituals, traditions, clothes and codes of conduct. As service provision is often geared towards society as a whole, services tend to overlook the cultural differences and needs of ethnic groups. This means that access to culturally appropriate respite or home care provision is reduced. Awareness of appropriate services and activities can also be limited due to different approaches to care and sense of responsibility and increased language barriers.

At the end of life

As a society we do not talk about death and dying:

> 'most of us find it hard to engage in advance with the way in which we would like to be cared for at the end of life.'

> *End of Life Care Strategy,*
> *Department of Health, 2008*

Most people do not discuss their own preferences for end of life care with their partner or family. Only around one third of the general public have discussed death and dying with anyone. End of life care for individuals with dementia should be well planned for with an inclusive care plan. This should consider all aspects of care including end of life care wishes and wants and should consider religion, advance directives, spiritual needs, cultural background, language and communications, symptom and pain management, family and friends, education and counsel and after death care. Health and support workers who work in care homes should familiarise themselves with the Gold Standard Framework. The Gold Standard Framework was developed to improve end of life experience for all individuals. Three key themes of the Gold Standard Framework (GSF) care homes work are:

- pre-planning
- improved communication
- improved team working.

LO3 Understand the importance of working in a person centred way and how this links to inclusion

In this section we will consider the importance of working in a person centred way and think about how this links to inclusion. Person Centred Planning was first developed in the 1980s by John O'Brien, Connie Lyle O'Brien, Beth Mount, Jack Pearpoint, Marsha Forest and Michael Smull. It was an approach that came from working in ways that enabled people – children and adults – to move out of special segregated places such as schools, hospitals, day and residential care institutions and into a mainstream arena. These were primarily schools and communities. A person centred approach was developed to help a person who has been disempowered to get the appropriate support to live the life they want.

Person Centred Planning is built on the values of inclusion and looks at the types of support an individual with dementia needs to be included and involved within their community. Person centred approaches offer an alternative to traditional types of planning which are based upon the medical model of disability. The medical model is orientated towards assessing need, allocating services and making decisions for people. This tends to be about doing for or doing to the individual with dementia. Instead, person centred planning is rooted in the social model and aims to empower people who have traditionally been disempowered by 'specialist' or segregated services by handing power and control back to them.

3.1 Explain how current legislation and government policy supports person centred working

There are sets of legislation and government policy that set out to support a person centred approach. This is because it is imperative that individuals receive care that is tailored to their needs. Therefore it is important that certain procedures are observed to make sure that individual needs are met and that individuals are central to care planning. This is so that they feel that they are actively involved in their own care.

Personalisation agenda

Personalisation is an approach to social care where 'every person who receives support, whether provided by statutory services or funded by themselves, will have choice and control over the shape of that support in all care settings' (Department of Health, 2011). The personalisation agenda tends to be underpinned by direct payments and personal budgets whereby individuals can fashion their own care packages rather than receiving a generic care plan that may not take into account individuals' care needs, preferences and of course cultural differences. However, there are concerns that certain groups, where lack of capacity may be an issue, may not fully benefit from this approach, in particular individuals with dementia. This approach is driven by an element of self-assessment.

Direct payments

Direct payments are a government initiative that was set up in 1996 and implemented in 1997. Direct payments are a resource that set out to give choice, freedom and scope for individuals to be responsible for shaping and paying for their social care. Direct payments are an important milestone in empowering disabled people and their rights towards living an independent life that they choose to live.

Mental Capacity Act 2005

This Act provides a statutory framework for acting and making decisions on behalf of individuals who lack the mental capacity to do so themselves. It introduced a set of laws to protect these individuals and ensure that they are given every chance to make decisions for themselves. The Act came into force in 2007. Deprivation of Liberties and Safeguarding are co-existing law.

Disability Discrimination Act (1995)

This states that a disabled person must not be treated any less fairly but equally to an able bodied person.

Health and Social Care Act 2008

This Act established the Care Quality Commission (CQC). The CQC remit is to protect and promote the rights of people using the health and social care service in England. The CQC regulates the provision of quality care. The CQC took over the roles carried out by the Healthcare Commission, Commission for Social Care Inspection and the Mental Health Commission in March 2009.

www.cqc.org.uk

The Equal Pay Act 1970 (amended 1984)

This Act says that women should be paid the same as men when they are performing the same role and carrying out the same work as men. The work is rated through a job evaluation scheme.

Race Relations Act 1976 (amended 2000)

This Act states that everyone must be treated fairly regardless of their race, nationality, or ethnic or national origins.

Human Rights Act 1998

This covers many different types of discrimination, including some that are not covered by other discrimination laws. Rights covered by the Act can only be used against a public authority, for example a local council or the police force and not a private company. Nevertheless, court decisions on discrimination usually take into account what the Human Rights Act would cover in relation to the case.

The National Dementia Strategy

This key document provides a strategic framework within which local services can deliver quality improvements and address health inequalities. The strategy provides advice, guidance and support for service providers and the third sector. It also provides practice based commissioners with information for planning, development and monitoring of services. The National Dementia Strategy also offers information for the creation and management of quality health and social care services aimed at individuals with dementia with the view to inform expectations and improve access to information and support.

Evidence activity

 Legislation and policies

This activity sets out to test how you think current legislation and government policy supports person centred working.

1. Why do we need laws to protect individuals with dementia?

2. What is person centred care?

3. How does the law promote person centred care?

3.2 Explain how person centred working can ensure that an individual's specific and unique needs are met

It is often assumed that when an individual receives a diagnosis of dementia the result is all 'doom and gloom', when in fact there is still a person who has rich and fulfilling life left to lead. Person centred care planning adopts a **holistic** approach, which means understanding the whole person. This includes, physical health, emotional, sexual, social, intellectual, mental and spiritual wellbeing. A person centred care approach considers all these needs as interrelated. By this we mean that if an individual's mental health is poor it may impact on physical health. An individual needing care has a heritage, history and an identity. Overlooking the requirement to adopt a person centred approach can be detrimental to the quality of care that is delivered.

Key terms

Holistic is seeing or observing the whole.

3.3 Describe ways of helping an individual's carers or others understand the principles of person centred care

Including an individual's carers or significant others in assessing needs and writing care plans can assist in understanding and delivering the principles of person centred care. This can often help carers see past the jargon of person centred care and understand what the term means. This approach outlines and explains the notion of person centred care and introduces the reasons for working with partnerships or external agencies when carers are finding it difficult to cope. Carers may be experiencing fear and anxiety or may be seeking solutions for particular problems. These negative aspects of caring can sometimes be overcome by including carers in the person centred care assessment. Furthermore, it may be appropriate to write a person centred care plan for carers or any significant others in that they may require respite or access to resources such as benefits, finance and technology.

Case Study

3.2 Sara

Sara is a 58-year-old woman who has recently received a diagnosis of dementia. She regularly attends dementia cafes, day centres and visits a memory clinic on a regular basis where she feels comfortable talking about areas of her life where she feels she needs support. As a result she has employed a personal assistant who provides support on an everyday basis and accompanies her on day trips out to art galleries and shopping. Sara also enjoys painting landscapes, which she does with the support of her personal assistant and her friends. Sara also enjoys her yoga classes and has recently become involved in a committee that aims to provide activities for people who have recently received a diagnosis of dementia and their families. Sara is feeling much happier now she has answers to some of the questions that were upsetting her before and that she has now access to resources that have improved her quality of life. Sara has lost one stone since her diagnosis due to her new exercise regime and is getting on much better with her partner Diane.

1) In what ways are Sara's person centred care assessments working for her?

2) What are the consequences of this on her holistic health?

3) In what ways do you think you could apply these techniques in your work setting?

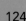

Evidence activity

 Helping understand the principles of person centred care

This activity sets out ways of helping an individual's carers or others understand the principles of person centred care.

1. What are the principles of person centred care?
2. What are the barriers often encountered by carers in seeking care and support to suit needs?
3. How does person centred care involve the carer?

3.4 Identify practical ways of helping the individual with dementia maintain their identity

There are numerous ways that can help individuals with dementia maintain their identity. This can be done physically and socially.

Physically

As individuals we all have a different sense of style; the clothes and shoes we wear are very important to our self identity. The way we organise our rooms and bedrooms also reflects our sense of who we are. Therefore for individuals with dementia the same applies. The bedroom may be arranged with homely items that denote aspects of the individual's identity. In other rooms around the home aspects of the local area such as pictures of surrounding areas, local occupations and objects can reinforce identity.

Socially

When interacting with individuals with dementia it is important to use their name and direct communication towards them in a reassuring manner. It is important to consider their cultural and ethnic background so that their diverse needs can be met. This person centred approach recognises a person's unique identity.

Evidence activity

 Practical ways of helping

This activity helps you identify practical ways of helping the individual with dementia maintain their identity.

1. Why is it important to maintain identity?
2. What are the physical aspects of identity?
3. What are social aspects to identity?

Assessment Summary DEM 310

Your reading of this unit and completion of the activities will cover the concepts of equality, diversity and inclusion that are fundamental to person centred care practice.

To achieve the unit, your assessor will require you to:

Learning Outcomes	Assessment Criteria
1 Understand the concept of diversity and its relevance to working with individuals who have dementia	**1.1** Explain what is meant by the terms • diversity • anti-discriminatory practice • anti-oppressive practice See evidence activities 1.1, pages 116 and 117
	1.2 Explain why it is important to recognise and respect an **individual's heritage** See evidence activity 1.2, page 118
	1.3 Describe why an individual with dementia may be subjected to discrimination and oppression See evidence activity 1.3, page 118
	1.4 Describe how discrimination and oppressive practice can be challenged See evidence activity 1.4, page 119
2 Understand that each individual's experience of dementia is unique	**2.1** Explain why it is important to identify an individual's specific and unique needs See evidence activity 2.1, page 119
	2.2 Compare the experience of dementia for an individual who has acquired it as an older person with the experience of an individual who has acquired it as a younger person See evidence activity 2.2, page 120
	2.3 Describe how the experience of an individual's dementia may impact on **carers** See evidence activity 2.3, page 120
	2.4 Describe how the experience of dementia may be different for individuals • who have a learning disability • who are from different ethnic backgrounds • at the end of life See evidence activity 2.4, page 121
3 Understand the importance of working in a person centred way and how this links to inclusion	**3.1** Explain how current legislation and government policy supports person centred working See evidence activity 3.1, page 123
	3.2 Explain how person centred working can ensure that an individual's specific and unique needs are met See case study 3.2, page 124
	3.3 Describe ways of helping an individual's **carers** or **others** understand the principles of person centred care See evidence activity 3.3, page 125
	3.4 Identify practical ways of helping the individual with dementia maintain their identity See evidence activity 3.4, page 125

DEM 313 Equality, diversity and inclusion in dementia care practice

What are you finding out?

Diversity describes many numerous types of things or people as part of something. For individuals with dementia in a health and social care setting it is important for diversity to be a main focus. This is because of the different age groups, different cultures and different ways of thinking. A helpful way of understanding diversity is to think about the last time you were in the town or city centre. Think about how diverse the people were that you saw: did you see people of different cultures; did you see tall people or small people; did you see any older people or disabled people? Do you know any vegetarian or gay people? The elements that make up diversity are present in many areas of the community. Diversity is all around us on our way to work, when we go shopping and on the television. When we go about our daily life we all form part of a diverse society. Indeed the term 'Diversity' is the name of a famous dance group because it reflects diversity through various age groups, different cultures and even height differences. Diversity means that as people come from a variety of backgrounds and have different life experiences so not everyone's views and tastes will be identical. If we use this model, we can begin to recognise diversity by identifying differences and working with this in our everyday living.

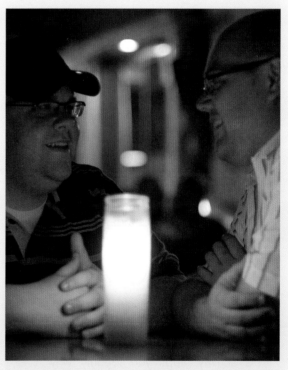

Figure 4.5

Reading this unit and completing the activities will allow you to:

- Understand that each individual's experience of dementia is unique

- Understand the importance of diversity, equality and inclusion in dementia care and support

- Be able to work in a person centred manner to ensure inclusivity if the individual with dementia

- Be able to work with others to encourage support for diversity and equality

LO1 Understand that each individual's experience of dementia is unique

Each person was born into different families, different circumstances, made different choices and had different life experiences. Difference is what makes each and every one of us unique. Not everyone with dementia is the same.

1.1 Explain why it is important to recognise and respect an individual's heritage

It is important to recognise and respect an individual's heritage so that you can give person centred care. This is important so that their needs and wishes can be met. An individual's heritage refers to an individual's culture, history and personal experiences and is unique to them. As a support worker it is vital that you recognise and respect an individual's heritage as this will provide insight into some of the key areas that can be considered when thinking about a person's quality of life and what makes them feel happy or upset. Understanding an individual's heritage considers how past life experiences could cause their own prejudices and therefore facilitates a deeper perceptive and sensitive approach to improving an individual's quality of life. It also provides clues into behaviour that we find challenging.

Evidence activity

 Thinking about heritage

This activity helps you identify why it is important to recognise and respect an individual's heritage.

1. What does heritage mean?
2. What clues can help you understand an individuals' heritage?
3. Who could you speak with about an individuals' heritage?
4. Why would you need to recognise and respect an individual's heritage?

1.2 Compare the experience of dementia for an individual who has acquired it as an older person with the experience of an individual who has acquired it as a younger person

Older people are generally more accepting of care, and service provision could be more likely to be orientated towards the issues that an older person with dementia may encounter. An older person may be of pensionable age and have no work commitments. Younger people with dementia are classified as being under 65 years old.

Physically, older people will experience aspects of the natural ageing process such as visual impairment or problems with eyesight, hearing impairment, limited mobility or dexterity and are perhaps a little more accepting of the changes that they are experiencing physically.

Evidence activity

 Compare and contrast experiences

This activity helps you compare the experience of dementia for an individual who has acquired it as an older person with the experience of an individual who has acquired it as a younger person.

	Older person	Younger person
What are the similarities?		
What are the differences?		
What are common difficulties?		
How are they overcome?		

Socially, older people may not have the types of social networks that a younger person may have. Families and friends may also be elderly and have conditions and illnesses that impair them. Older people tend to be socially excluded and do not participate in everyday outings like younger people may do.

1.3 Describe how the experience of dementia may be different for individuals:

With a learning disability

It is considered important to understand what the term 'learning disability' actually means.

A learning disability includes the presence of:

'A significantly reduced ability to understand new or complex information, to learn new skills (impaired intelligence), with;

A reduced ability to cope independently (impaired social functioning); which started before adulthood, with a lasting effect on development.'

(*Valuing People*, 2001)

The experience of dementia may be different for people who have a learning disability because some of the symptoms, characteristics and behaviours of learning difficulties are similar to that of some dementias. This can mean that the onset of dementia can be diagnosed later than that of an individual who has not got a learning disability. A person may already have underlying cognitive impairment, and difficulty with living skills. Individuals with learning disabilities are prone to health problems and can also display and experience symptoms similar to those of dementia. These can be compounded and diagnosis missed through communication difficulties in conveying what they may be experiencing. In addition, the subtle changes may also be missed because of staff turnaround as carers or support workers change frequently.

For people with learning difficulties communication can often be improved by using simpler language and avoiding technical terms. People with learning difficulties often benefit from incorporating signs and symbols such as Makaton into their communication techniques. Incorporating this type of communication aid can assist in understanding others and help others to understand them. It can be very frustrating when individuals, their carers and staff find it difficult to understand or 'get through'. By considering and adopting alternative communication strategies individuals with learning disabilities can communicate more effectively.

Different ethnic backgrounds

Ethnic background or ethnicity is where a person identifies with one another through a shared language, faith or religion, specific geographical location or ideology. This unification is often characterised by food, rituals, traditions, clothes and codes of conduct. Therefore it is important to consider how the diverse needs of individuals with dementia are met.

Case Study

1.3 Mrs Aadab

Mrs Aadab is an 83-year-old Muslim woman originally from Pakistan. She prays at least five times a day. She carries out ritual washing before she prays. She does not read but recites verses of the Holy Quran. She eats Halal food and because of her religious beliefs does not eat pork. Mrs Aadab always covers her head and wears her clothes in bed. She does not eat with knives and forks but prefers to eat with her fingers. She looks forward to seeing her family who visit her in her residential care home every week. Mrs Aadab fasts in the month of Ramadan. All Muslims must fast in this month where they must not eat from just before dawn to sunset in the evening. However, there are exceptions, usually where people are mentally or physically unwell. Sometimes she doesn't fast because of her ill health. Other times when she feels well she will fast.

1) In what ways may Mrs Aadab's experience of dementia be different?

2) What are the consequences of Mrs Aadab's ethnic background on her care plan?

3) In what ways do you think you could support Mrs Aadab's needs?

At the end of life

Providing support for individuals with dementia who are at the end of their lives is a very challenging role. This aspect of care can be improved by ensuring advance directives have been sought so that the needs and wishes of the dying person can be carried out. This type of planning also should consider emotional and physical comfort as well as spiritual or religious needs. This is an important time where your knowledge of the person through life story work and personal experience can really benefit end of life care. Creating an appropriate environment is vital. Talking about death and dying is often shied away from but being prepared and planning ahead with the individual with dementia and their family and friends presents positive outcomes. It's normal to think that people do not want to talk about end of life matters because traditionally it has been a taboo subject, but often when we approach this subject in a calm and sensitive manner it can be very reassuring because needs and wishes can be taken into account. For example, playing favourite music may soothe the person and make them feel safe. Understanding that each individual is unique and recognising distractions can create an environment that is calm and peaceful and appropriate for them. It is also important to recognise that individuals with dementia who have learning disabilities or severe communication difficulties may find it difficult to express pain or mask other symptoms. This can lead, for example, to the under-treatment of pain and/or the overuse of evasive interventions such as artificial feeding or hydration in the latter stages of life.

1.4 Describe how the experience of an individual's dementia may impact on carers

Families and carers of individuals with dementia play an essential role in helping to look after them by assisting with and helping them maintain their independence. Families and carer's achieve this through providing ongoing support, care and help with day-to-day tasks for individuals who would otherwise struggle to manage on a day-to-day basis. As we have seen throughout this book individuals with dementia often present other contributing factors that require specific care such as physical ailments and other symptoms concurrent with the natural ageing process. Fulfilling this role may be compounded and present additional effort if the carer is elderly or has poor health themselves. In addition, the mental and intellectual challenges families and carers often encounter, such as repetitive questioning, frustrations, orientation, spatial awareness, aphasia and agnosia, can be very stressful and mentally arduous. Carers also face a set of behavioural and interpersonal challenges such as difficulty walking, failing to recognise, hitting out, forgetting to turn the gas off, sleep disturbance and restlessness.

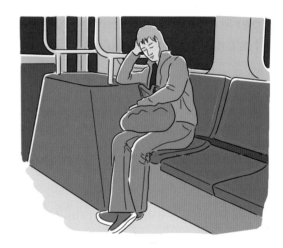

Figure 4.6 Carers have to cope with many pressures.

Family carers of individuals with dementia often become carers very gradually and move step by step into the role as a full time carer. Therefore carers' mental health and wellbeing can often be affected. For example carers can often experience senses of loss or bereavement not only for the person they are caring for, but also for aspects of themselves and who they are. There are a number of reasons why these issues can creep in. Below are some examples of what a carer may feel and experience:

- resentment
- loss and bereavement of the former person
- loss of self identity
- reduced sociality
- isolation
- experience of negative emotions, such as guilt, anger, embarrassment, disgust
- loss of financial stability and work
- stress
- fatigue
- concern
- love and hope
- helplessness
- a feeling of being overwhelmed.

Key terms

Aphasia is an acquired communication disorder that impairs a person's ability to process language, but does not affect intelligence.

www.aphasia.org

Agnosia is an inability to recognise objects, faces or surroundings.

Dysarthia is difficulty in speaking where speech becomes unclear, as is often the case after a stroke.

Evidence activity

 1.4 Supporting carers

What kind of information could you give carers to support them? Where/how could you direct them to gain more support and information?

LO2 Understand the importance of diversity, equality and inclusion in dementia care and support

In this section we will consider the importance of diversity, equality and inclusion in dementia care and support and the legislation and policy that upholds it.

2.1 Describe how current legislation, government policy and agreed ways of working support inclusive practice for dementia care and support

There are sets of legislation and government policy that set out how to support a person centred approach. This is because it is imperative that individuals receive care that is tailored to their needs. Therefore it is important that certain procedures are observed to make sure that individual needs are met and that individuals are central to care planning. This is so that they feel that they are actively involved in their own care.

Personalisation agenda

Personalisation is an approach to social care where 'every person who receives support, whether provided by statutory services or funded by themselves, will have choice and control over the shape of that support in all care settings' (Department of Health, 2011). The personalisation agenda tends to be underpinned by direct payments and personal budgets whereby individuals can fashion their own care packages rather than receiving a generic care plan that may not take into account individuals' care needs, preferences and of course cultural differences. However, there are concerns that certain groups, where lack of capacity may be an issue, may not fully benefit from this approach, in particular individuals with dementia. This approach is driven by an element of self-assessment.

Direct payments

Direct payments are a government initiative that was set up in 1996 and implemented in 1997. Direct payments are a resource that set out to give choice, freedom and scope for individuals to be responsible for shaping and paying for their social care. Direct payments are an important milestone in empowering disabled people and their rights towards living the independent life that they choose to live.

2.2 Describe the ways in which an individual with dementia may be subjected to discrimination and oppression

There are a number of ways that an individual with dementia may be oppressed and these are often unintentional. Not allowing enough time to communicate, doing things for a person rather than allowing time for them to do for themselves, dignity during personal care, using labels and having stereotypical views can all oppress individuals with dementia.

Discrimination is more clearly defined in terms of legal frameworks and policies that address issues such as race, sexuality, gender, religion, class, ethnicity and human rights. An individual with dementia could be subject one or more of these types of discrimination.

Research and investigate

Discrimination

This activity will help you analyse the ways in which an individual with dementia may be subjected to discrimination and oppression.

1. What key pieces of legislation spring to mind when you think about discrimination?

2. What recent news stories have you heard about discriminatory practice?

Explain the potential impact of discrimination on an individual with dementia

Discrimination impacts on individuals with dementia in negative ways. In particular, this is because individuals with dementia are very vulnerable. Discrimination can affect how people feel about themselves and their dignity. Dignity is concerned with how people feel, think and behave in relation to self-worth and the way they think about others. To treat someone with dignity is to treat them in a way that values them and is respectful. In care situations, dignity may be promoted or diminished in a number of ways.

Evidence activity

Potential impact of discrimination

This activity will help you explain the potential impact of discrimination on an individual with dementia.

1. How does legislation aim to protect people, in particular individuals with dementia?

2. What areas do you identify with?

3. If this were to happen to you how would these circumstances make you feel?

4. What could be the possible outcome for you, your family and your health?

When dignity is ignored people feel bad about themselves, out of control and distressed. They may lose confidence and feel humiliated, embarrassed or ashamed. Able-bodied people who face discrimination can challenge their oppressors because they have the skill sets and resources to do so. However, individuals with dementia do not have the opportunities to challenge discrimination as they are vulnerable. Individuals with dementia may socially withdraw or not feel comfortable participating in activities. This is not good for mental wellbeing and can lead to heightened senses of low self-esteem and perhaps a more serious mental health issue such as depression.

Analyse how diversity, equality and inclusion are addressed in dementia care and support

Every person that works in a health and social care role must demonstrate their ability to promote equality, diversity and challenge discrimination against individuals with dementia, their carers, families and colleagues. This can be achieved by adopting the social model and developing an inclusive approach that means being reflective about what you do, how you engage at work and thinking about how your attitude may affect your work. Think about stereotypical views and the way that these views affect the ways people interact with individuals with dementia. Then consider that these types of interaction may be seen by others who could follow your direction. On the other hand if you label or stereotype people and are prejudiced about people then you can rightly be accused of being discriminative.

Labels are descriptive words that are used to describe another person or their characteristics. Street language would call this 'name calling'. For example, older people are often referred to as 'old dear', 'cute', 'blue rinse'. Labelling or name calling is dangerous because it infers negative connotations and can blur the positive aspects of individual's characteristics. The 'blue rinse' may have been instrumental in the Normandy Landings in the Second World War and received an OBE for her work there. Similarly, she could have been a Prime Minister.

It is all too easy to stereotype people. Stereotyping assumes that all people from certain groups are all the same. Of course, individuals with dementia may share one or two similar characteristics, as do nurses or families. However if we take for granted that every person in the group is the same then we lose sight of their individuality.

Attitudes can also be dismissive or patronising, particularly towards an individual's beliefs, values or cultural background. This may then come across as being unconcerned and nonchalant about their individual needs and be detrimental to your ability to fulfil your duty of care and support. Instead, maintain a positive attitude and refrain from talking about your prejudices regardless of differences. You need to be inclusive and accepting of diversity. Adopting a warm, welcoming and respectful approach towards everyone shows people that you value them for who they are.

You can get to know the people that you work with by talking with them and their friends and families. In the same vein, get to know your colleagues and the other professionals that you work with and know the individuals with dementia that you all support and care for. Seek to contribute to life stories and care plans. Read and digest care plans and assessments and do not be afraid to ask questions. Learn about the things that people like and dislike. What are their cultural backgrounds and beliefs; what are their experiences? Increasing and adding breadth to your understanding of why people think the way they think and behave the way they behave will provide you with a rich and resourceful toolkit. This toolkit will provide you with a variety of useful tools that will enable you to support individuals with dementia appropriately. It will also allow you to make sure that you assist the people that you support in exercising their rights and meet their needs.

In terms of workplace policy, make sure that you are familiar with these procedures and that you observe policies that promote equality and diversity. It is good to be familiar with the documents that relate to the minimum standards of and codes of practice. These can be found on the Care Quality Commission website (www.cqc.org.uk). As a health and social care worker you owe individuals with dementia 'a duty of care', equally they can expect a reasonable standard of care from all workers.

Evidence activity

 Addressing issues of diversity, equality and inclusion

This activity will help you analyse how diversity, equality and inclusion are addressed in dementia care and support. List the elements that could indicate discrimination within different contexts, providing solutions and ways of challenging discrimination in the lowest row. The final column is there for you to add your own ideas or thoughts of where you think discrimination may have occurred.

	Race, religion and ethnic background	Age, gender,	Sexuality and personal relationships	Family	Your own ideas
Legal • List legislation					
Social • Communication • Food and drink					
Physical • Environment • Room layout					
Solutions and ways of challenging					

LO3 Be able to work in a person centred manner to ensure inclusivity of the individual with dementia

A person centred approach to care and support is fundamental to all aspects of health and social care. A person centred approach was developed to help people who have been disempowered – for whatever reason – to live the life that they want and to get the right support in doing this. Therefore the personal attributes, individuality, needs, aspirations and what makes people tick must be at the heart of what we do to support individuals and promote their wellbeing. As we discussed in Chapter 1 DEM 201 Section 2.2, as well as thinking about the physiological problems an individual with dementia may face it is particularly important that we observe a social model approach. Tom Kitwood's famous words claimed that we should 'see the person first not the dementia'.

(**Tom Kitwood** was the Leader of Bradford Dementia Group and Senior Lecturer in Psychology at the University of Bradford.)

By seeing the person first and not the dementia, Kitwood argued that we should take account of the whole person. This means that as well as taking into consideration the physical and chemical aspects of dementia affecting the brain that may affect the way a person thinks and acts, you must also see that this will be unique to them. The way a person reacts and responds to the changes that their dementia will bring will also be affected by the ways in which we behave and interact with individuals with dementia. As a support worker it is particularly important to ensure that an individual with dementia can retain their sense of identity, confidence and dignity. It is crucial that an individual's personhood, heritage and all of the things that make them who they are and makes them unique are observed.

3.1 Demonstrate how to identify an individual's uniqueness

In understanding that every individual has a distinct personality and characteristics it is vital to demonstrate how to identify an individual's uniqueness. One way of doing this should be care planning and assessment. This can be carried out with individuals with dementia and their carers,

family members and friends. Activities such as life story work are a useful vehicle that capture important information about a person's identity, supporting the person in maintaining their individuality and independence wherever possible. This can be achieved by focusing on what the person can do rather than what they cannot do. In order to understand the perspective of individuals it is often useful to try and understand how they themselves make sense of their situation.

Evidence activity

3.1 Understanding individuality

List the words that you use for certain activities or everyday tasks.

- food
- shopping
- bathing.

What is your bedtime routine?

What would you do if you could not do these things?

What things do you dislike?

3.2 Demonstrate how to use life experiences and circumstances of an individual who has dementia to ensure their inclusion

The experiences and circumstances of an individual who has dementia can be used effectively to ensure their inclusion in a variety of ways. As discussed previously we can use a variety of techniques and approaches to identify how life experiences and circumstances form distinctive characteristics making everyone unique. Life experience can be usefully thought of as a patchwork quilt. If we think of all of our experiences and circumstances as being patches of our identity then we can see how everyone's is different. The use of various tools to elicit this information from individuals with dementia can form part of the activities schedule. Family and friends are also valuable sources of information. You could also do your own research into specific occupations, places, food or even music. This information can be usefully integrated into the

Evidence activity

(3.2) Be able to work in a person centred manner to ensure inclusivity of the individual with dementia

This activity will help you show you can identify an individual's uniqueness. It will also help you understand how to use the life experiences and circumstances of an individual who has dementia to ensure their inclusion, maintain their dignity and incorporate this into daily life.

	Explain why this is important	Who else can help. • Team workers • Family and friends • Other practitioners	Action taken	Result/ reflection	Next steps
What makes them happy?					
What are signs of distress or unhappiness?					
Food and drink					
Religion and spiritual beliefs					
Cultural background					
Past jobs and roles					
Achievements					
Significant others					
Hobbies					
Music, TV, reading					
Activities					

Evidence activity

3.2 Making a bedroom sign

This activity will demonstrate how to use the life experiences and circumstances of an individual who has dementia to ensure their inclusion.

Information gathered from 'life story work' forms an integral part of creating the bedroom sign. Images tend to show the individual with dementia as they are currently. Due to cognitive changes recognition may be a problem, therefore a favourable image or picture should be used.

To locate an appropriate image here are some questions or thought that you might find useful.

- What were/are your favourite pastimes?
- Have you any memorable times/people/animals/places?
- What is your preferred name?

This exercise allows the good practices of life history to be integrated in to the environment. In doing this we are:

- Creating a sense of ownership and dignity.
- Aiding recognition and improved orientation.
- Collecting personal and relevant information for meaningful interactions and promoting a person centred care approach.

List any information below that you would give to someone who was making your bedroom sign.

1.
2.
3.
4.
5.
6.

physical and social environment. This could be in topics discussed, using fragrances or even pieces of furniture and objects. Discussing topics using physical objects or sensory elements can heighten the inclusion felt.

Remember not to have discussions and talks with only your colleagues when supporting people with dementia. Always include the person with dementia and make them the centre of what you do. Here are a few useful ways of including people.

- Remember to put the person at the centre of your conversations and never talk over their head when you are with another member of staff.
- Include the person in the conversation, talking about topics that are relevant and interesting to them.
- Explain carefully what you are doing when you are supporting them with personal care, demonstrate active listening by mirroring, and tailor activities and expectations to their personal abilities.

3.3 Demonstrate practical ways of helping an individual with dementia to maintain their dignity

Dignity is concerned with how people feel, think and behave in relation to self-worth and the way they think about others. To treat someone with dignity is to treat them in a way that values them

Evidence activity

3.3 Personal dignity

List five things that would diminish your dignity.

1.
2.
3.
4.
5.

List five ways that someone you care about could make you feel better.

1.
2
3
4
5

and is respectful. In care situations, dignity may be promoted or diminished in a number of ways. When dignity is ignored people feel bad about themselves, out of control and distressed. They may lose confidence and feel humiliated, embarrassed or ashamed. The following list highlights some of the areas that you could think about when maintaining an individual's dignity.

- Physical environment
  - orientation
  - food and drink
  - clothing
  - colour/contrast
  - room layout.
- Social Environment
  - work culture
  - attitudes and behaviour
  - personal care
  - shared language
  - name
  - specific words/names
  - personal care.

There are no set lists as to what you should do to when maintaining dignity, therefore the list above provides you with practical ways that will help you do this.

 3.4 **Demonstrate how to engage and include an individual with dementia in daily life**

We all need to feel valued and included and able to engage or fit into daily life. Our routines are important to us because we have roles in life that mean that we do things for ourselves and others that are meaningful. The ways in which an individual with dementia may feel valued, included and able to engage in daily life can have an effect on their mental wellbeing and physical health. The ways in which individuals can engage in daily life will depend on lots of different factors and may fluctuate or change from one day to the next. One day may be better than another. Every individual has different interests, roles and talents. In the same vein, there are activities and pastimes that some people do not like. We have different likes and dislikes because everyone is unique. It is important to understand what roles individuals like to take, their pastimes and interests, in order to assist them in participating in daily life. For example, one person may like setting the table whilst another may like gardening or tidying up. Understanding what makes people tick and helping them to achieve and realise those interests can help them feel included and valued in daily life.

Evidence activity

3.4 Engagement and inclusivity

This activity will help you demonstrate how to engage and include an individual with dementia in daily life.

Think of three daily tasks that an individual with dementia may be able to do:

- in their own home to improve dexterity
- in a care home to work as a team
- in hospital to generate conversation.

LO4 Be able to work with others to be able to encourage support for diversity and equality

As a health and social care and support worker it is important that as well as striving to encourage support for diversity and equality you encourage colleagues and others to do the same. Others could mean practitioners that you work with on a daily basis. The following list outlines who these others could be:

- care worker
- colleague
- manager
- social worker
- occupational therapist
- GP
- speech and language therapist
- physiotherapist
- pharmacist
- nurse
- psychologist
- Admiral nurses
- Independent Mental Capacity Advocate
- Community Psychiatric Nurse

- dementia care advisors
- advocate
- support groups.

Work with others to promote diversity and equality for individuals with dementia

It is very important that we promote diversity and equality for individuals with dementia when working with others. This can be done by communicating and sharing individual's diverse backgrounds with others who also may offer support. It is vital that new information is shared whilst observing confidentiality.

Evidence activity

4.1 Working with others to promote diversity and equality

This activity will help you work with others to promote diversity and equality for individuals with dementia.

1. Give a ten minute presentation to your colleagues about what diversity and equality means to you and get feedback about what it means to them.

2. Create a poster for the staff room highlighting what diversity and equality means.

4.2 Demonstrate how to share the individual's preferences and interests with others

There are a number of ways that an individual's preferences and interests can be shared. First and foremost this should be done via a carefully compiled care plan that documents preferences and interests specific to the individuals that you work with. These should include triggers and descriptive behaviours resulting from any incidents that may have occurred. This document can be consulted and offer insights into an individual's background and heritage. Second, by adopting a social model approach; this involves including every person, such as the cooks and chefs in the kitchen, the maintenance team and housekeepers. They also may be able to share preferences and interests with you. Actively supporting individuals to do things encourages individuals to do as much for themselves as possible. This helps to maintain independence and physical ability and encourages people with disabilities to maximise their own potential and independence.

Evidence activity

4.2 Sharing preferences and interests

This activity will help you demonstrate how to share an individual's preferences and interests with others.

- Create a person centred planning process that maps where a person would like to be in the future.

- Organise a meeting with key team players to discuss their views and encourage conversation to provide a variety of views.

Liaise with the individual with dementia and their families and friends.

4.3 Explain how to challenge discrimination and oppressive practice of others when working with an individual with dementia

In order to challenge discrimination and the oppressive practice of others it is useful to listen to the views of others and individuals with dementia. It is also useful to familiarise yourself with the correct channels that you should use should you ever find yourself in a situation where you need to report any incidents that you consider to be discriminative or oppressive. Talking about equality and diversity in everyday work practice can alert your colleagues and encourage them to think about their behaviour and the language that they may use at work.

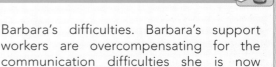

Case Study

 Barbara

Barbara has moderate stage dementia and her communication abilities have declined considerably over the last two weeks. She is experiencing significant difficulties in finding words. As a result her support workers have started talking loudly over her and using derogatory terms to describe

Barbara's difficulties. Barbara's support workers are overcompensating for the communication difficulties she is now experiencing.

1) In what ways is Barbara being discriminated against?

2) In what ways could you challenge these types of behaviour?

Further resources:

www.dhcarenetworks.org.uk

Assessment Summary DEM 313

Your reading of this unit and completion of the activities will provide you with knowledge, understanding and skills for those who provide care or support to individuals with dementia in a wide range of settings. The unit covers the concepts of equality, diversity and inclusion, which are fundamental to person centred approach.

To achieve the unit, your assessor will require you to:

Learning Outcomes	Assessment Criteria
1 Understand that each individual's experience of dementia is unique	**1.1** Explain why it is important to recognise and respect an **individual's heritage** See evidence activity 1.1, page 128
	1.2 Compare the experience of dementia for an individual who has acquired it as an older person with the experience of an individual who has acquired it as a younger person See evidence activity 1.2, page 128
	1.3 Describe how the experience of dementia may be different for individuals: • who have a learning disability • who are from different ethnic backgrounds • who are at the end of life See case study 1.3, page 129
	1.4 Describe how the experience of an individual's dementia may impact on **carers** See evidence activity 1.4, page 131

Learning Outcomes	Assessment Criteria
2 Understand the importance of diversity, equality and inclusion in dementia care and support	**2.1** Describe how current legislation, government policy and agreed ways of working support inclusive practice for dementia care and support See research and investigate activity 2.1, page 132
	2.2 Describe the ways in which an individual with dementia may be subjected to discrimination and oppression See research and investigate activity 2.2, page 132
	2.3 Explain the potential impact of discrimination on an individual with dementia See evidence activity 2.3, page 132
	2.4 Analyse how diversity, equality and inclusion are addressed in dementia care and support See evidence activity 2.4, page 133
3 Be able to work in a person centred manner to ensure inclusivity of the individual with dementia	**3.1** Demonstrate how to identify an individual's uniqueness See evidence activity 3.1, page 134
	3.2 Demonstrate how to use life experiences and circumstances of an individual who has dementia to ensure their inclusion See evidence activities 3.2, pages 135 and 136
	3.3 Demonstrate practical ways of helping an individual with dementia to maintain their dignity See evidence activity 3.3, page 136
	3.4 Demonstrate how to engage and include an individual with dementia in daily life See evidence activity 3.4, page 137
4 Be able to work with others to encourage support for diversity and equality	**4.1** Work with **others** to promote diversity and equality for individuals with dementia See evidence activity 4.1, page 138
	4.2 Demonstrate how to share the individual's preferences and interests with **others** See evidence activity 4.2, page 138
	4.3 Explain how to challenge discrimination and oppressive practice of **others** when working with an individual with dementia See case study 4.3, page 139

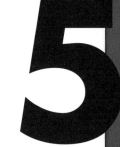

Rights, Choices and Risks
DEM 211 Approaches to enable rights and choices for individuals with dementia whilst minimising risks

What are you finding out?

It is a common preconception that when an individual has received a diagnosis of dementia they have no capacity or skills in making choices or decisions about their life and their wishes and needs for the future. This is not true. Rather individuals with dementia should be encouraged to talk about their likes and dislikes so that we can offer support to help them realise their goals and desires. This unit provides you with knowledge, understanding and skills that are required to promote individuals' rights and choices whilst minimising risk. Learning Outcomes 3 and 4 must be assessed in the workplace environment.

Reading the unit and working through the activities will enable you to:

• Understand key legislation and agreed ways of working that ensure the fulfilment of rights and choices of individuals with dementia while minimising the risk of harm

• Understand how to maintain the right to privacy, dignity and respect when supporting individuals with dementia

• Support individuals with dementia to achieve their potential

• Be able to work with carers who are caring for individuals with dementia

LO1 Understand key legislation and agreed ways of working that ensure the fulfilment of rights and choices of individuals with dementia while minimising risk of harm

1.1 Outline key legislation that relates to the fulfilment of rights and choices and the minimising of risk of harm for an individual with dementia

The Health and Social care sector has to adhere to legislation and policy to ensure that the work and care they perform is lawful and to ensure that individuals' rights and choice are fulfilled. There are various legal frameworks that are important and that you are legally required to observe in your everyday work. The following outlines some of the key legislation.

Key legislation

Mental Health Act 2007

This Act amends the Mental Health Act 1983 (the 1983 Act) and the Mental Capacity Act 2005 (MCA). The Act is mainly concerned with the circumstances in which a person with a mental disorder can be detained for treatment for that disorder without his or her consent. The main purpose of the legislation is to ensure that people with serious mental disorders which threaten their health or safety or the safety of the public can be treated irrespective of their consent where it is necessary to prevent them from harming themselves or others.

The following are the main changes to the 1983 Act made by the 2007 Act:

- definition of mental disorder so that a single definition applies throughout the Act
- criteria for detention
- broadening of professional roles who can intervene
- nearest relative: the provisions now include civil partners amongst the list of relatives.

Amendments to the Mental Capacity Act 2005

The 2007 Act makes a number of amendments to the Mental Capacity Act 2005 (MCA). The main change is to provide for procedures to authorise the deprivation of liberty of a person in a hospital or care home who lacks capacity to consent to being there. This is the introduction of the Deprivation of Liberty Safeguards.

Mental Capacity Act 2005

This Act provides a statutory framework for acting and making decisions on behalf of individuals who lack the mental capacity to do so themselves. It introduced a set of laws to protect these individuals and ensure that they are given every chance to make decisions for themselves.

Mental Capacity and Deprivation of Liberty Safeguards 2005

Deprivation of Liberties and Safeguarding are co-existing law. Individuals who have a disorder or a disability of the mind such as dementia or a learning disability may lack the mental capacity to seek and consent to the treatment and care they need. In these cases, individuals still have the right to be cared for in a way that does not limit their rights and freedom of actions. However, in some cases individuals who lack capacity to make informed decisions need to be deprived of the liberty so that appropriate treatments and interventions can be administered to protect and safeguard their health and wellbeing. For this group of people Deprivation of Liberty Safeguards provides the legal framework that safeguards them from harm. When it is identified that a person who lacks mental capacity is, or is at risk of being deprived of their liberty an application must be submitted to a supervisory body for the authorisation of the deprivation of liberty. The Code of Practice for Deprivation of Liberty Safeguards must be read alongside the Mental Capacity Act Code of Practice, as they both apply. There is no standard set of criteria that constitutes what a deprivation of liberty may be but here are some examples:

- staff and care staff having control over all of the decisions in an individual's life
- not being allowed to leave the care home or hospital where one lives
- friends, family and carers not being able to visit.

Deprivation of Liberty Safeguarding (DOLS) applies to people in England and Wales.

Adults with Incapacity (Scotland) Act 2000

This Act provides legal protection for individuals who live in Scotland. It was introduced to protect the finances and property of vulnerable adults over the age of 16 who lack the capacity to make informed decisions. This can be due to a physical condition or a mental disorder. It allows others to make decisions on behalf of the adults, subject to safeguards. The main groups covered with this legislation are people with dementia, learning disabilities, an acquired brain injury, chronic and severe mental health illness and sensory impairment. The Act's aim is to put the person central to the focus of the solutions. For example, a person with dementia may be able to make decisions about their everyday life but not their finances. In such cases, just a financial intervention may be necessary but the Act provides a framework that may combine welfare and financial measures.

For further information see
http://www.scotland.gov.uk/Resource/
Doc/217194/0058194.pdf

Safeguarding Vulnerable Groups Act 2006

The Safeguarding Vulnerable Groups Act 2006 was passed as a result of the Bichard Inquiry arising from the Soham murders. This was when two school children were murdered by Ian Huntley who was a caretaker at their school. The Inquiry investigated the way background checks are carried out when recruiting people to work with vulnerable groups. Recommendation 19 of the Inquiry Report argued for a legal framework that would vet all individuals who want to work or volunteer with children or vulnerable adults.

http://www.isa-gov.org/default.
aspx?page=321

Carers (Equal Opportunities) Act 2004

The Carers (Equal Opportunities) Act ensures that carers are able to take up opportunities that people without caring responsibilities often take for granted. For example, the right to work, study or take part in leisure activities. It is intended to provide a firm foundation for better practice by councils and the health service. It builds on existing legislation and support for carers by:

- placing a duty on local authorities to ensure that all carers know that they are entitled to an assessment of their needs
- placing a duty on councils to consider a carer's outside interests (work, study or leisure) when carrying out an assessment
- promoting better joint working between councils and the health service to ensure support for carers is delivered in a coherent manner.

http://www.direct.gov.uk/en/
CaringForSomeone/CarersRights/
DG_4018108

Disability Discrimination Act (1995)

This states that a disabled person must not be treated any less fairly but equally to an able bodied person.

Health and Social Care Act 2008

This Act established the Care Quality Commission (CQC). The CQC remit is to protect and promote the rights of people using the health and social care service in England. The CQC regulates the provision of quality care. The CQC took over the roles carried out by the Healthcare Commission, Commission for Social Care Inspection and the Mental Health Commission in March 2009.

www.cqc.org.uk.

The Equal Pay Act 1970 (amended 1984)

This Act says that women should be paid the same as men when they are performing the same role and carrying out the same work as men. The work is rated through a job evaluation scheme.

Race Relations Act 1976 (amended 2000)

This Act states that everyone must be treated fairly regardless of their race, nationality, or ethnic or national origin.

Human Rights 1998

This covers many different types of discrimination, including some that are not covered by other discrimination laws. Rights covered by the

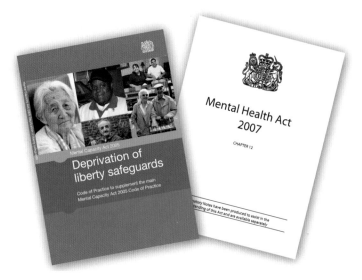

Figure 5.1 It is important to be aware of key legislation.

Act can only be used against a public authority, for example a local council or the police force, and not a private company. Nevertheless, court decisions on discrimination usually take into account what the Human Rights Act would cover in relation to the case.

There are sets of legislation and government policy that set out to support a person centred approach. This is because it is imperative that individuals receive care that is tailored to their needs. Therefore it is important that certain procedures are observed to make sure that individual needs are met and that individuals are central to care planning. This is so that they feel that they are actively involved in their own care.

Personalisation agenda

Personalisation is an approach to social care where 'every person who receives support, whether provided by statutory services or funded by themselves, will have choice and control over the shape of that support in all care settings' (Department of Health 2011). The personalisation agenda tends to be underpinned by direct payments and personal budgets whereby individuals can fashion their own care packages rather than receiving a generic care plan that may not take into account individuals' care needs, preferences and of course cultural differences. However, there are concerns that certain groups, where lack of capacity may be an issue, may not fully benefit from this approach, in particular, individuals with dementia. This approach is driven by an element of self-assessment.

Direct payments

Direct payments are a government initiative that aims for individuals to be responsible for shaping and paying for their social care. Direct payments are an important milestone in empowering disabled people and their rights towards living an independent life that they choose to live.

Research and investigate

 Acts and policies

Think about the needs of the people you support and the type of service your workplace provides. Make a list of the acts and policies that you think apply in your work setting. Talk your answer through with your manager or employer.

1.2 **Describe how agreed ways of working relate to the rights of an individual with dementia**

The term 'agreed ways of working' sets out how your employer wants you to work. To implement 'agreed ways of working' in the health and social care sector means following a care plan that manages daily care, takes into consideration the rights of an individual and makes reference to relevant legislation and policy as best practice. You must listen to and respect the individual's choices and input into the decision-making process. It is an individual's right to be proactive in the decisions made about their care.

Evidence activity

1.2 Agreed ways of working

Think about the needs of an individual that you support and their care plan. Write down examples of where agreed ways of working recognise the rights and needs of the individual. Talk your answer through with your manager or employer.

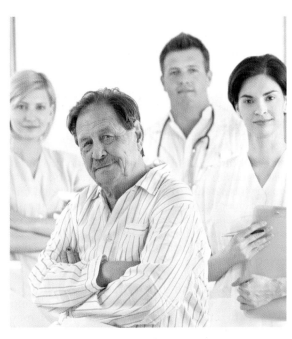

Figure 5.2 Different professions and roles work to agreed standards, policies and procedures – agreed ways of working.

1.3 Explain why it is important not to assume that an individual with dementia cannot make their own decisions

It is often assumed that once an individual has been diagnosed with dementia then there is little or no hope of leading a fulfilling life. In fact, the exact opposite is true if managed using an abilities approach. Good examples of how people with dementia can still lead a fulfilling and influential life can be found with organisations such as the Scottish Dementia Working Group (SDWG) who advocate the rights of people with a diagnosis of dementia. The organisation was founded and is run by individuals with a diagnosis of dementia. The SDWG have been very influential in policy making and funding allocation. However, perhaps the most important thing that people with dementia can tell us is about how services, support and technology can either assist or disempower individuals with dementia. The SWDG maintain that one of most disempowering issues that they face is the way that able bodied people constantly remind them of the things that they cannot do any more. The SWDG also explained that they felt that the negative aspects and debilitating progressive nature of the condition were often discussed between medical practitioners and family members as if they were not in the room. Therefore it is important to take into account that individuals who have dementia can still make decisions. Individuals with dementia need to feel part of the decision making processes that affect them and in some cases may affect other individuals with dementia and their carers.

Evidence activity

1.3 Decision-making

Write down five reasons why an individual can make decisions.

1.

2.

3.

4.

5.

1.4 Explain how the best interests of an individual with dementia must be included when planning and delivering care and support

It is important to consider the best interests of an individual when planning and delivering care plans. This could be in creative ways that provide methods by which individuals can be proactive in the compiling of their care plan. In adopting this approach we are being person centred and respecting an individual with dementia by considering their likes and dislikes. When an individual with dementia lacks capacity to make a decision, actions and decisions must be based on the person's best interests. Furthermore, the individual with dementia should still be involved in making decisions. People who know the person well, such as family, friends and care staff, can offer guidance. This can be done as an activity with family members and friends. Such decisions are known as **best interest decisions** and should where possible limit restrictions placed on the person. However it should be noted that capacity issues should be accounted for and a relevant risk assessment put in place to ensure the safety of individuals with dementia whilst facilitating positive risk taking.

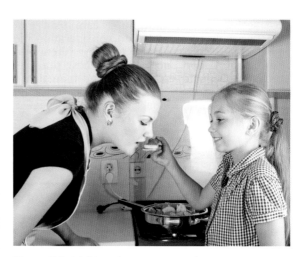

Figure 5.3 Making decisions together.

Key terms

Best interest decisions consider an individual with dementia's likes and dislikes and wishes and desires when planning and delivering care and support.

Evidence activity

1.4 Best interest decisions

Ask a manager to let you 'buddy' a work colleague when they are working with best interest decisions to plan and deliver care.

1.5 Explain what is meant by providing care and support to an individual with dementia in the least restrictive way

In providing care for individuals with dementia we need to think about offering care and support in the least restrictive way. It is important that the support and care you give assists individuals with dementia to perform everyday tasks such as eating, drinking, getting dressed and personal care issues but also that their choices and needs are recognised. The care and support offered also needs to facilitate positive risk taking whilst observing safeguarding. Sometimes an individual with dementia may be put into a care home so that they may be cared for properly. This may be done without their consent based on an assessment of their needs. However, despite being placed in care by the authorities, the individual with dementia has a legal right to exercise their rights and freedom within the institution. It is vital that we offer care and support in a least restrictive way so that we may help people maintain skills, independence and dignity while also obeying the law.

1.5 Providing care and assistance

Think about an individual who has recently moved into your care setting. List five areas where you think that they may need assistance in their everyday life.

1.

2.

3.

4.

5.

How can you support them in the least restrictive way?

LO2 Understand how to maintain the right to privacy, dignity and respect when supporting individuals with dementia

Individuals with dementia have the right to participate in work, leisure and educational activities. They also have the right to access information, knowledge and resources that assist them with everyday living and also to make decisions that may affect them. Individuals with dementia have the right to be treated fairly irrespective of age, gender, sexual orientation, religion or ethnic background. However, there may be instances when certain aspects of an individual's personal life and care may need intervention. Issues of confidentiality should be observed. While it may be necessary to discuss individuals' care needs it is not acceptable to talk about individuals with dementia in, for example, tea breaks. This breaks confidentiality and impacts on individuals' privacy and dignity and shows no respect. When such conversations need to take place a quiet room should be used. This room can also be used for other private conversations with family members. Personal records should be kept somewhere secure and the the relevant authority should be bestowed on staff for access. Conversations about people should never take place in front of an individual with dementia unless they are to be involved. Never talk about a person as if they are not there. Individuals with dementia should also have their personal space respected.

Staff should knock before entering a room. Where close monitoring or surveillance is needed then this should be done in the most unintrusive way.

2.1 Privacy and dignity

Imagine you were an individual with dementia. How would you feel if you kept having your privacy and dignity compromised?

2.1 Describe how to maintain privacy when providing personal support for intimate care to an individual with dementia

It is very important to maintain privacy when providing personal support for intimate care such as bathing, going to the toilet and dressing. When entering a room it is respectful to knock and perhaps say the name of the person you are going to support. This is also respectful of privacy as intimate care may be already being given. When removing clothes try and keep as much of their body covered as possible and try to keep doors closed. Try and learn the types of words that the individual is familiar with for private parts and going to the toilet. Always explain to the person what you are doing and keep a calm voice and manner. Giving support for intimate care can often mean dealing with unpleasant smells so it is important that you do not make reference to this. Open a door or a window and try and stay calm otherwise this can be very distressing. Often an individual may feel embarrassed about noise so singing or playing music can help to preserve dignity.

2.1 Privacy and support for intimate care

List three ways that you provide privacy and support when giving intimate care.

1.

2.

3.

2.2 Give examples of how to show respect for the physical space of an individual with dementia

It is important to show respect for the physical space of an individual with dementia to maintain privacy and dignity. It is important to knock before you enter a room. This shows respect for the individual with dementia and observes privacy within their physical space. This is also a place where intimate care may already be taking place. Respect for physical space can also be achieved by thinking about how they may want their environment to be and assistance can be offered in supporting individuals with dementia in creating a homely room. Their desired food and an appropriate time to eat it also shows respect. It is also important to show respect for physical space in terms of communication. It shows more consideration to maintain the same level of eye contact when communicating. When engaging with individuals with dementia it is important to consider the physical space between you. It is important not to assume and invade someone's space.

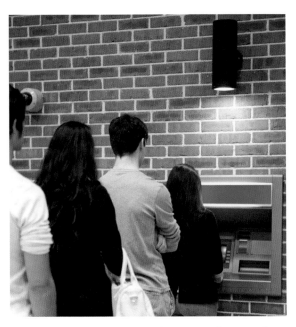

Figure 5.4 We must respect the personal space of a person with dementia. Consider how you would feel if the next person in this queue stood too close to you.

Evidence activity

2.2 Privacy

What ways could you show respect for the physical space for three different individuals with dementia?

Who could you talk to?

2.3 Give examples of how to show respect for the social or emotional space of an individual with dementia

It is important to consider the social and emotional wellbeing of individuals with dementia. This involves thinking about their social and emotional space by listening, learning and observing. Touch can be acceptable in some cultures, for example a hug can be comforting, whereas for other cultures this may not be appropriate. Showing respect for social and emotional space is about being person centred and understanding that all individuals are unique. Good tools for finding out about individuals are life story books, memory boxes, photographs, pictures and objects that relate to the individual you are supporting. Examples of social and emotional space are those that take the individual's heritage and life story into account:

- food
- pastimes
- spirituality
- room design
- music
- film.

Encourage them to express feelings, use a calm and interested tone of voice and interactive body language.

Evidence activity

2.3 Social environment

What tools would you use to understand an individual with dementia's likes and dislikes?

How could you use this information and incorporate it into the social environment?

2.4 Describe how to use an awareness of the life history and culture of an individual with dementia to maintain their dignity

The awareness of the life history and culture of an individual with dementia can maintain dignity because it provides information, knowledge and tools that assist in an understanding of their likes and dislikes. This level of understanding takes into consideration, for example, clothes, food, age and the past and future achievements individuals with dementia may still hope to realise. It also points to some of the experiences that individuals have lived and how these may have affected them on an emotional level. The awareness that individuals with dementia are unique and may have alternative ways of doing things preserves dignity as we respect who they are.

Time to reflect

2.4 Awareness

Imagine that your parents or partner did not know anything about you. What could they give you for your birthday? To eat for your tea? Where would they take you out for a special occasion?

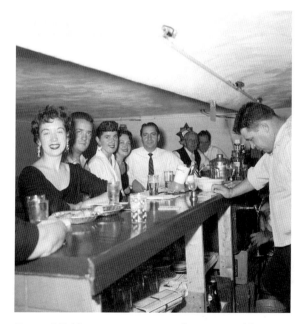

Figure 5.5 Have an awareness of a person's life history or culture.

2.5 Outline the benefits of knowing about the past and present interests and life skills of an individual with dementia

The benefits of knowing about past and present interests and life skills of individuals with dementia can inform us about future interactions and communications. The types of things that we are interested in shape how we live our daily lives. Past and present interests form part of our sense of inclusion and worthiness on a daily basis. Therefore, setting the table, folding napkins or laundry may be something one person likes to do whilst another likes tending to the garden or pot plants. Past and present experiences also shape the way we spend our leisure time. For example, some people may like to watch a film whilst others enjoy making things or painting. By knowing about people's past and present interests we can set goals and achievements whilst also being aware of not setting unrealistic targets for them.

Evidence activity

2.5 Past and present interests

This activity will give you an opportunity to think about ways of organising meaningful activities.

Write down a list of the current and past interests of three members of your family or friends.

In what ways did you learn about these interests?

How did you participate in such interests?

How has this information informed your decision-making?

LO3 Support individuals with dementia to achieve their potential

It is important to support individuals with dementia to achieve their potential. This ability approach provides physical and social environments that are accessible for people with dementia.

3.1 Demonstrate how the physical environment may enable an individual with dementia to achieve their potential

The physical environment plays a massive role in how individuals with dementia perform everyday tasks, orientate themselves and maintain skill sets. It is argued that the physical environment can in fact create disabilities when it is not sensitive to the needs of people with dementia.

Front door

A care environment can have many doors and entrance points. There needs to be a focal point that will be used for welcoming new service users, residents, their families and friends. This entrance should have adequate lighting that will trigger with movement. A welcome sign should be situated at eye level at around 1300mm.

Entrance hall

Coat and umbrella stands, a clock and seasonal calendar could be used. A fish tank could be placed here. There should be a clear and visible toilet sign; painting the toilet door in a way that is consistent throughout the care environment can help with orientation.

Corridors

It is a widespread assumption that people living with dementia mostly have problems with their memory. Whilst memory problems are a major symptom of dementia, people living with dementia also experience changes in the ways that they see or visualise their surroundings. Therefore the rooms and corridors need to be adequately lit. As you can see in the first image in Figure 5.7 the room is quite dark. This can make it difficult to see and presents problems for orientation while obstacles may hinder walking around.

For people who experience visual difficulties a change in surface colour can give the impression of a step or change of depth. This is because some areas of the brain that process information have been affected by dementia. This then leads to distortion or a misinterpretation of the carpet strip. When asking people to move over carpet strips or onto a change of floor surface the perceived step or depth can cause anxiety. If possible maintain a constant colour throughout. As you can see in the second picture in Figure 5.7 there is a constant colour below that presents a confident route into the lounge area. Shiny surfaces can give the impression of water. The image above shows how the shine may present significant challenges due to perhaps a fear of slipping.

Due to the changes in how the brain processes information it is important to think about how we can use colour to improve recognition. For example, if the chairs are of a similar colour to the floor. This could present a problem for someone sitting down as it could be difficult to set them apart from the floor. In the image below the chairs are of a colour that contrasts starkly with the floor. This helps seeing that there is a chair and may improve confidence in sitting down. Similarly, white table cloths, white napkins and white crockery could blend into one mass of colour making it difficult to distinguish between the plates and the table cloth. White crockery often hides lighter foods such as mashed potato, rice or fish pie. In Figure 5.7 we can see how the use of coloured crockery aids in making the food stand out much more clearly. You can see how it would be easy to overlook that there was a drink in the beaker. If possible use coloured beakers or if this is not possible then squash or cordial can assist with recognition as in the picture overleaf.

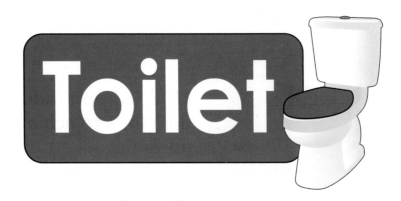

Figure 5.6 A clear and visible sign for a toilet.

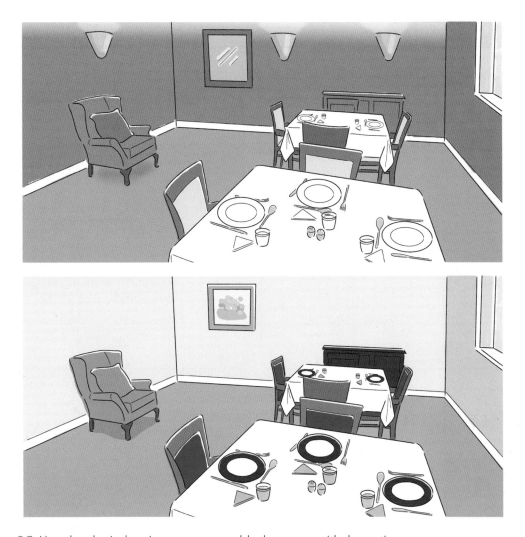

Figure 5.7 How the physical environment can enable the person with dementia.

Mirrors are useful for admiring reflections or fixing hair or make up, but for people living with dementia mirrors can be frightening or disturbing because sometimes the reflection may not be recognised. It is common for reflections to be mistaken for strangers, imposters or maybe a family member. Whilst mirrors can be useful it should be noted that mirrors can present potential problems. Instead, culturally relevant images can be used. Pictures of food draw attention to food in the dining area. This can aid with way finding, orientation, a sense of location and perhaps stimulate appetite. It is common to put pictures of landscapes and flowers on walls as means of decoration; however these types of images do not stimulate interaction or conversations. If we use pictures of people, places or objects that are meaningful then these can provide many more opportunities for discussion or distraction particularly in difficult moments.

Finding out about people's life history and what the images are could form part of your activity schedule. This can be further improved by using objects that reflect your residents' pasts. A seasonal clock showing the time, day and month may offer reassurance.

The corridors off the entrance hall are the initial routes that a new service user will take. The floor should be covered using a consistent colour. Patterns can present obstacles for people. Shiny and sparkly floors can give the impression of water or objects on the floor. There should be a clear colour contrast between the floor and the walls. This can be achieved by painting the skirting boards. Handrails should also be distinguished from the wall using contrasting coloured paint. A matt gloss can reduce shiny patches.

Evidence activity

(3.1) The importance of the physical environment

This activity will help you to understand how the physical environment may enable individuals with dementia to achieve their potential.

	Explain why this is important	What areas need improving?	How can they be improved?	What aspects of an indiividual's potential will be enhanced?	Who else can help? Team workers, family and friends
Living Room					
Dining Room					
Corridors					
Bedroom					
Toilets					
Other communal areas					

(3.2) Demonstrate how the social environment may enable an individual with dementia to achieve their potential

The social environment is a term that covers:

- communication skills
- positive approach
- relationship centred approach
- professional boundaries
- abilities focus
- whole team approach.

The social environment can be a negative place for individuals with dementia where it is understimulating. It can be boring, repetitive, noisy, disrespectful and often this can cause social withdrawal, apathy and behaviours we find challenging. It can cause individuals to disengage and lose interest. The social environment can be enhanced by having a respectful and courteous manner and through the introduction of activity groups such as reading, painting or gardening. This type of social interaction can assist people to interact with others because the social environment is pleasant and one that provides a variety of activities that are meaningful and challenging.

Social environment

Fill in the table below to help you understand how the social environment can influence experiences of dementia.

	Explain why this is important	What else can help? Team workers, family and friends
Noise		
Boredom		
Repetitive Behaviour		
Communication		
Food		

3.3 Support an individual with dementia to use their abilities during personal care activities

It is good practice to encourage individuals with dementia to use their abilities with all tasks including personal care. Often support workers become tempted to do things for people, usually because they feel that they are doing the right thing by 'doing to' or 'doing for'. It can also be that there is so much to do and that time is an issue, in that individuals with dementia may take longer to do something that may take only a few moments to do yourself. Therefore waiting for an individual to undo their trousers may seem an eternity when support staff are aware that they have many other jobs that they ought to be doing. When we do too much for people or overcompensate for what we perceive to be their disabilities we often diminish confidence, reduce sense of dignity and as a result skill sets are lost and depression can occur. This is because a person who can do something is not provided with the correct channels to demonstrate their capabilities, exercise their potential and exhibit competence.

Evidence activity

3.3 Supporting individuals with dementia to use their abilities during personal care

This activity will give you an opportunity to think about ways of supporting individuals with dementia to use their abilities during personal care.

Write down a list of the current and past needs of personal care.

Demonstrate what you might need to do to create the right setting for personal care.

3.4 Explain how the attitudes of others may enable an individual with dementia to achieve their potential

The attitudes of others around individuals with dementia can have a huge influence on their ability to achieve their potential. Person centred means seeing the person before the dementia and understanding their dislikes, likes, past and current interests. A person centred approach also means that we understand that every person is unique and should be treated with respect and dignity. This is instead of being task orientated, that is, thinking about the jobs and tasks you have to perform on a daily basis rather than how you conduct yourself when giving care and support. A patient, reassuring and attentive approach can instil a sense of hope where individuals with dementia look forward to interacting with you because of the ways in which you listen and assist in everyday tasks. Reaching one's potential is not merely about winning gold medals but rather how we achieve on a day-to-day basis.

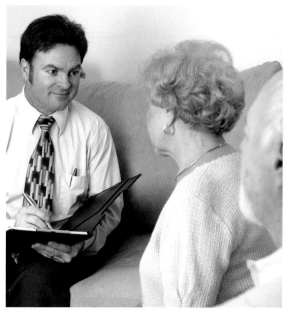

Figure 5.8 It is important to include and consult with carers. They are often the 'experts' in the care of the person with dementia.

Evidence activity

3.4 Attitudes and achieving potential

This activity will give you an opportunity to think about the ways that other's attitudes enable individuals with dementia to reach their potential.

Produce a poster for display in the staff room entitled 'Attitudes and achieving potential', which describes skills and approaches needed to enable people to reach their potential.

LO4 Be able to work with carers who are caring for individuals with dementia

As a health and social care worker it is important to be able to work with carers who are caring for individuals with dementia. In what follows we will consider some of the issues that you may encounter.

4.1 Identify some of the anxieties common to carers of an individual with dementia

Carers of individuals with dementia often feel an array of emotions. Whilst carers have strong attachments to the people they care for, and love their family members dearly, they may also experience negative emotions. As a health and social care worker it is important to recognise these so that you may offer support and direction for resources or other information they may need. It is common for carers to experience senses of grief/loss due to perceived loss of the person they used to know. It is also common for carers to feel a loss of the life that they used to live. Carers can also be stressed through providing support for repetitive behaviours, not being recognised and dealing with the deterioration of skill sets or language. Carers can also feel isolated as it is common for social withdrawal to occur without realising it as socialising is not often an option anymore. Carers can also feel resentment due to the new lifestyle that has begun for them since their loved one started to dement. Carers may also be frightened and scared about what is happening. Even feelings of guilt can envelope carers as they realise that they cannot look after their loved one for much longer and how this may impact on their future. It is important to recognise that feeling these types of emotions and anxieties is normal. On balance it is a natural way of dealing with matters, but we should remember that every carer is unique too and that they will need support and guidance. It is common for carers to feel anxieties as they may feel like they are the only ones experiencing such things. Try and offer comfort and reassurance by showing that you recognise such anxieties, and provide them with information or just listen.

Evidence activity

 4.1 Understand the anxieties of carers

This activity will help you to understand the anxieties of carers.

List five reasons why carers may be anxious.

1.
2.
3.
4.
5.

 ## Outline the legal rights of the carer in relation to an individual with dementia

There are numerous pieces of legislation and policies that set out to inform carers of their legal rights in relation to the care of individuals with dementia. Carers' needs should be addressed in accordance with the Carers of Disabled Children (2000) and Carers (Equal Opportunities) Act (2004). The assessments should consider the psychological and psychosocial health of the carer and provide interventions, support and training to provide them with the support and tools they need to maintain a good standard of health. In addition to welfare, carers also have rights that cover a whole range of issues in relation to future care. Legislation covers issues such as:

- Advance Decisions/Directive
- Lasting Power of Attorney
- Community of Practice.

Evidence activity

 4.2 Legal rights of carers

This activity will give you the opportunity to be aware of the legal rights of carers.

Speak to your manager about the different types of legislation and how these affect the rights of carers.

4.3 ## Involve carers in planning support that enables the rights and choices and protects an individual with dementia from harm

Health and social care professionals should involve carers in all aspects of care and planning. Individuals with dementia should always be considered as having the capacity to make decisions until proved otherwise. Involving carers in enabling rights and choices also assists in assessing needs and wishes and also the individual's capacity. Adopting a person centred approach is important and good communication skills are essential. There are a number of resources that can be accessed free. 'Caring with confidence' is an online resource offered by the NHS which informs carers of their rights and the services available to them and helps develop their advocacy and networking skills. In planning support that enables rights and choices it is essential that carers are involved so that their needs are also considered and assessed.

Evidence activity

4.3 Involving carers in planning and support that enables rights and choices of individuals with dementia

This activity will give you an opportunity to think about ways of involving carers in planning and support that enables rights and choices of individuals with dementia

- What area of care and support are you planning?
- Who will you consult?
- What tools will you use?
- How will you communicate?

4.4 Describe how the need of carers and others to protect an individual with dementia from harm may prevent the individual from exercising their rights and choices

Often in the caring role it is common for carers to overcompensate for perceived disabilities and diminishing skill sets. This is not intentional. In doing things for people and helping them too much it is common for individuals with dementia to 'give up' or 'stop trying' because everything has been done for them. Think about when people do things for you, for example a parent picking up dirty washing. This can often lead to children not having to think about picking things up and taking them to the wash basket or the washing machine. The result is a loss of an opportunity to learn to maintain skills sets and the ability to perform an everyday task. The busy schedule of caring for individuals with dementia can also mean that it is often quicker to do the task yourself. It may take an individual with dementia 30 minutes to dress or over an hour to eat their breakfast. If a carer intervened it would take minutes but the individual with dementia should have the opportunity to do things for themselves. Carers' own insecurities, when they perceive others looking and making judgements, can also lead to embarrassment and excuses being made on behalf of the individual with dementia. Diminishing language skills can also lead carers to believe that the person they care for has no capacity to make decisions which may lead to decisions being made on their behalf. Instead an abilities approach is more useful, although a little more time consuming, and advocates rights and choices.

Evidence activity

 Exercising rights and choices

This activity will give you an opportunity to demonstrate how the need of carers and others to protect an individual with dementia from harm may prevent the individual from exercising their rights and choices.

1. List why you may rush or do something for another person.
2. Provide a way of carrying out the same role but now encouraging people to do things a little more for themselves.

4.5 Demonstrate how a carer can be supported to enable an individual with dementia to achieve their potential

A carer probably knows lots about the interests, likes and dislikes of the individual with dementia and by having the right support carers can enable the people they care for to reach their potential. It's very important that carers are aware of the resources that offer such support as soon as possible. This information can be found locally in GP surgeries, libraries and other community groups. Information can also be found online. A carer will need to know where to find information and be made aware of funding or benefits that they may be entitled to. It is important as a health and social care worker that you have good communications skills, that you are a good listener to carers' needs and that you can recognise their needs. By carrying out assessments you can better understand the areas that carers need support in. For example, personal care, finance, driving or health and nutrition.

Evidence activity

 Achieving potential

This activity will give you an opportunity to demonstrate how a carer can be supported to enable an individual with dementia to achieve their potential.

Ask a manager to let you buddy with a senior work colleague at a planning meeting with carers.

In what areas does the individual with dementia need support?

What can be done to support the carer?

Assessment Summary DEM 211

Your reading of this unit and completion of the activities will have provided you with knowledge, understanding and skills required to promote individuals' rights and choices whilst minimising risk. Learning Outcomes 3 and 4 must be assessed in the workplace environment.

To achieve the unit, your assessor will require you to:

Learning Outcomes	Assessment Criteria
1 Understand key legislation and agreed ways of working that ensure the fulfilment of rights and choices of individuals with dementia while minimising risk of harm	**1.1** Outline key legislation that relates to the fulfilment of rights and choices and the minimising of risk of harm of individuals with dementia See research and investigate activity 1.1, page 144
	1.2 Describe how agreed ways of working relate to the rights of an individual with dementia See evidence activity 1.2, page 145
	1.3 Explain why it is important not to assume that an individual with dementia cannot make their own decisions See evidence activity 1.3, page 145
	1.4 Explain how the best interests of an individual with dementia must be included when planning and delivering care and support See evidence activity 1.4, page 146
	1.5 Explain what is meant by providing care and support to an individual with dementia in the least restrictive way See evidence activity 1.5, page 147
2 Understand how to maintain the right to privacy, dignity and respect when supporting individuals with dementia	**2.1** Describe how to maintain privacy when providing personal support for intimate care to an individual with dementia See evidence activity 2.1, page 147
	2.2 Give examples of how to show respect for the physical space of an individual with dementia See evidence activity 2.2, page 148
	2.3 Give examples of how to show respect for the social or emotional space of an individual with dementia See evidence activity 2.3, page 148
	2.4 Describe how to use an awareness of the life history and culture of an individual with dementia to maintain their dignity See time to reflect 2.4, page 149
	2.5 Outline the benefits of knowing about the past and present interests and life skills of an individual with dementia See evidence activity 2.5, page 149

Learning Outcomes	Assessment Criteria
3 Support individuals with dementia to achieve their potential	(3.1) Demonstrate how the physical environment may enable an individual with dementia to achieve their potential See evidence activity 3.1, page 152
	(3.2) Demonstrate how the social environment may enable an individual with dementia to achieve their potential See evidence activity 3.2, page 153
	(3.3) Support an individual with dementia to use their abilities during personal care activities See evidence activity 3.3, page 153
	(3.4) Explain how the attitudes of others may enable an individual with dementia to achieve their potential See evidence activity 3.4, page 154
4 Be able to work with carers who are caring for individuals with dementia	(4.1) Identify some of the anxieties common to carers of an individual with dementia See evidence activity 4.1, page 155
	(4.2) Outline the legal rights of the carer in relation to an individual with dementia See evidence activity 4.2, page 155
	(4.3) Involve carers in planning support that enables the rights and choices and protects an individual with dementia from harm See evidence activity 4.3, page 155
	(4.4) Describe how the need of carers and others to protect an individual with dementia from harm may prevent the individual from exercising their rights and choices See evidence activity 4.4, page 156
	(4.5) Demonstrate how a carer can be supported to enable an individual with dementia to achieve their potential See evidence activity 4.5, page 156

DEM 304 Enable rights and choices of individuals with dementia whilst minimising risks

What are you finding out?

This unit can be read in conjunction with Unit 211 (page 141). You will understand how we implement key legislation to support the rights and choices of people with dementia as well as protecting them from harm. This also involves the support of others. We will also understand how we maintain the privacy and dignity of the person whilst ensuring their rights and choices are upheld.

Reading through the unit and completing the activities will ensure that you:

• Understand key legislation and agreed ways of working that support the fulfillment of rights and choices of individuals with dementia while minimising risk of harm

• Are able to maximise the rights and choices of individuals with dementia

• Are able to involve carers and others in supporting individuals with dementia

• Are able to maintain the privacy, dignity and respect of individuals with dementia whilst promoting rights and choices

LO1 Understand key legislation and agreed ways of working that support the fulfilment of rights and choices of individuals with dementia while minimising risk of harm

We have learnt in the unit DEM 211 that the health and social care sector must work within certain legislation. This legislation applies to all sectors of health and social care, whether it is a public organisation like the NHS or a private care home. The rights of people under the law remain the same, wherever they may be. The law reflects the changing needs and circumstances of people and therefore it is important to have an understanding of how each law supports people's rights in different ways.

1.1 **Explain the impact of key legislation that relates to the fulfilment of rights and choices and the minimising of risk of harm for an individual with dementia**

The key legislation we are looking at is:

1. Human Rights Act 1998
2. Mental Capacity Act 2005
3. Mental Health Act 2007
4. The Disability Discrimination Act 1995
5. Safeguarding Vulnerable Groups Act 2006
6. Carers (Equal Opportunities) Act 2004.

1. Human Rights Act 1998

This legislation **upholds the rights** of all people as citizens, regardless of race, gender, age, **disability (which includes dementia)**. The Human Rights Act is very important for people with mental health problems because it **protects** their rights and legislates (upholds the law) against discrimination, **abuse** and denial of access to services open to other people.

Some human rights include:

- the right to life
- freedom from torture and degrading treatment

- the right to liberty
- the right to respect for private and family life
- freedom of thought, conscience and religion, and freedom to express your beliefs
- freedom of expression
- freedom of assembly and association
- the right to marry and to start a family
- the right not to be discriminated against in respect of these rights and freedoms
- the right to peaceful enjoyment of your property
- the right to an education
- the right to participate in free elections.

If any of these rights are not upheld people also have **the right to it being dealt with through the law.**

2. Mental Capacity Act (MCA) 2005

This Act provides a statutory framework for acting and making decisions on behalf of individuals who lack the mental capacity to do so themselves. It introduced a set of laws to protect these individuals and ensure that they are given every chance to make decisions for themselves. All professional people have a duty to comply with the Act. There should be procedures in your place of work which help you to understand and work through the MCA.

The Act has been in force since 2007 and applies to England and Wales. It is estimated that about two million people in England and Wales lack capacity to make decisions for themselves.

- **Rights and choices** – it empowers people to make decisions for themselves, whenever possible.
- **Protects from harm** – it places vulnerable people at the centre of the process and takes their preferences and choices into account, rather than assuming they do not have a 'voice'.

If a person with dementia is assessed as 'lacking capacity' then any decision or action made on their behalf must be in their best interest.

Key terms

Capacity is having sufficient memory to retain insight into a situation and to be able to use this insight to make informed decisions.

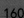

Before acting in a person's best interests we must test their capacity, and always remember that we are assessing capacity to make specific decisions; it is not good enough to make a general statement that someone lacks capacity. There are key principles to follow to protect the person:

- Presume capacity unless you have evidence to show they do not have capacity (this is done by using a prescribed test). Do not assume because the person has dementia they automatically lack capacity. Indeed they may have the capacity to make many decisions.

- If the person does lack capacity to make a certain decision, consider the least restrictive option. For example, if the person does not have the capacity to understand the danger of crossing the road, this does not mean they cannot leave the building. The least restrictive option might be to accompany them.

- Remember that unwise decisions do not mean the person lacks capacity. I may own one hundred pairs of shoes and decide I need another pair – this does not automatically mean I lack capacity.

- Always involve the person in any decisions. Think about what we have learnt about person centred care and communication skills to enable you to ensure a person centred approach.

- Make the decision about the person in their best interest, not that of anyone else. Although family and friends' views and rights are important, we must protect the person from harm or coercion and so we must always try to understand what the person would want if they had full capacity. Equally, the role of family and friends is crucial as they may know what is important, but we must always weigh up 'best interests'.

The 2007 Act makes a number of amendments to the Mental Capacity Act 2005 (MCA). The main change is to provide for procedures to authorise the deprivation of liberty of a person in a hospital or care home who lacks capacity to consent to being there. This is the introduction of the Deprivation of Liberty Safeguards.

Mental Capacity and Deprivation of Liberty Safeguards 2005

The Deprivation of Liberty Safeguards provides the legal framework that safeguards vulnerable individuals from harm. The new provisions create a set of statutory safeguards that, when necessary, make it lawful to deprive an incapacitated person of their liberty. When it is assessed that a person who lacks mental capacity is, or is at risk of, being deprived of their liberty an application must be submitted to a supervisory body for the authorisation of the deprivation of liberty. The Code of Practice for Deprivation of Liberty Safeguards must be read alongside the Mental Capacity Act Code of Practice, as they both apply. There is no standard set of criteria that constitutes what a deprivation of liberty is, and in some circumstances it may be a 'restriction' of liberty. It will depend on the nature, frequency, and intensity of the deprivation.

Examples might be:

- staff and care staff having control over all of the decisions in an individual's life

- not being allowed to leave the care home or hospital where one lives

- friends, family and carers not being able to visit.

The Deprivation of Liberty Safeguarding (DOLS) applies to people in England and Wales.

If you work in a care home or hospital, you must familiarise yourself with the policies and procedures for DOLS. If, for example, a person with dementia is trying to leave the ward or care home, you must consider:

- How can I intervene and de-escalate this situation and prevent risk of harm?

- If the person insists on leaving, what powers do I have to detain them – what are their rights?

- What can I do if the person does leave?

- What steps would I need to take to ensure we manage this situation in the future?

3. Mental Health Act (MHA) 2007

This Act amends the Mental Health Act 1983 (the 1983 Act), and is a legal framework in which a person can be detained in hospital for assessment and treatment of their mental health without their consent. The main purpose of the legislation is to ensure that people with serious mental disorders which threaten their health or safety or the safety of the public can be treated where it is necessary to prevent them from harming themselves or others. People in these situations will lack capacity and insight into their situation and to minimise '**risk of harm**' require urgent support. People can be detained in hospital under two sections of the Act:

1. **Section 2 - Detention for assessment in hospital**

   Under Section 2 of the MHA, someone can be detained in hospital for assessment for a maximum of 28 days. If the medical professionals feel that more time is needed after this for further assessment, they can detain the person for another 28 days. Peoples' rights are protected because an Approved Mental Health Practitioner or the person's nearest relative has to ask for someone to be detained. Two doctors have to recommend using a section of the Act and one of those has to have specialist knowledge of mental health.

2. **Section 3 – Detention for treatment in hospital**

    Section 3 of the act is used when someone is to be detained in hospital for treatment, initially for six months. After this time, the section may be renewed for a further six months, and then for a year at a time. The process is the same as for detaining someone for mental health assessment under Section 2 except that the doctors must confirm there is appropriate treatment available for the person in hospital.

The MCA and the MHA also make provision for special advocates (Independent Mental Capacity Advocates and Independent Mental Health Advocates) who are appointed to support the person when difficult decisions need to be made in the person's best interests and they may not have relatives to support them.

People also have the **right to appeal** if they feel that they should not be detained in hospital. This is done in a Mental Health Act Tribunal, which like a court, is chaired by a judge. This is to protect the rights of the person to ensure whether they should or should not be detained against their will. The judge and a specialist panel make a decision once all the supporting evidence is heard. The detained person is also able to attend the tribunal.

4. Disability Discrimination Act 1995 (DDA)

From 1 October 2010, **The Equality Act** replaced most of the Disability Discrimination Act (DDA). However, the Disability Equality Duty in the DDA still applies. The spirit of both Acts remains the same, to ensure by law that a person with a disability must not be treated any differently because of their disability.

The Equality Act 2010 aims **to protect disabled people and prevent disability discrimination**. It provides **legal rights** for disabled people in the following areas:

*   Employment – that people with a disability have the right to be considered for employment.
*   Education – that people with a disability have the right to an education.
*   Access to goods and services and facilities – that people with a disability have the right

to enjoy goods services and facilities, like shops and social clubs.

*   Buying and renting land and property.

The Act also protects those who are associated with a person with a disability, and this includes family and friends who are carers.

5. Safeguarding Vulnerable Groups Act 2006

The Safeguarding Vulnerable Groups Act 2006 was passed as a result of the Bichard Inquiry arising from the Soham murders. The Act introduced new requirements for those who work with children and vulnerable adults to be registered. This provided a framework for a vetting and barring scheme for those people who are unsuitable and **pose a risk to children and vulnerable people.**

It is likely that when you have applied for a job in health or social care you have been required to complete a form which enables the employing authority to ask for a criminal records check. In most jobs in public services, when you work with people, you will be told that you are not exempt from the Rehabilitation of Offenders Act and that the police authority will disclose any previous convictions to your potential employer. **This is to protect vulnerable people from risk of harm.**

6. Carers (Equal Opportunities) Act 2004

This Act ensures that carers have the same opportunities that people without caring responsibilities have. The Carers (Equal Opportunities) Act came into force in April 2005. It places certain responsibilities on local authorities to ensure that carers know they have a right to an assessment of their needs. This not only protects the rights of carers but can help the

Research and investigate

 Policies and procedures

Look at the policies and procedures at your place of work. How much information is available for staff, people with a disability like dementia, and family carers? How could you improve this? You could produce a poster, for example, outlining the rights of people.

person with dementia if the carers themselves are supported. The principle of this act is to ensure that the rights of carers are not ignored or that carers as a resource are not 'take for granted'.

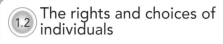 Evaluate agreed ways of working that relate to rights and choices of an individual with dementia

Agreed ways of working not only include the types of legislation we have described. It also includes the policies and procedures of your organisation. There are many ways that your place of work may describe agreed ways of working. You may have a code of practice, or a statement of values, or a 'residents' charter'. As part of your induction as a new member of staff

Evidence activity

1.2 The rights and choices of individuals

Consider the learning outcome for this unit. Ask yourself some questions:

- How do you as an individual and the organisation you work in fulfil the rights and choices of people with dementia and ensure minimum risk of harm? The rights and choices of the person should be reflected in their care plan, personal profile and life history. How much notice do you take of these things?

- Are these documents working tools or are they sat in a drawer and not looked at?

- How up to date are your risk assessments? Does everyone have an awareness of the risks and needs of the person they support? Remember, people are constantly changing.

- When was the last time you discussed practice issues – do you use handover sessions, or training events or reflective practice as opportunities to evaluate how you approach issues of rights and risks?

- Is there relevant educational material available for both staff and carers?

you may have had to think about the aims and objectives of the service you offer.

All these ways of working are statements of intent – they tell us how you are going to apply the principles of the key legislation. As an individual and an organisation you will be measured by regulatory bodies like the Care Quality Commission (CQC) who regulate how well a service supports the people in its care.

■ Research and investigate

1.2 Rights and choices

Use a search engine to find the CQC website, or ask to see a copy of the CQC document 'Essential Standards of Quality and Safety'. Read Part 2 outcomes 1, 4, 7. Design an information leaflet which explains the rights of people with dementia in your service.

1.3 Explain how and when personal information may be shared with carers and others, taking into account legislative frameworks and agreed ways of working

There are a variety of legislation and codes of practice that relate to information sharing in health and social care. These include The Codes of Practice for the Mental Health Act and Mental Capacity Act, NHS Records Management, The Human Rights Act, codes of practices for nurses and social workers and the Data Protection Act 1998.

The main principles include the person's right to **confidentiality** and that if information is to be shared the person is informed about how and why this information is being shared. Everyone has a duty under the Data Protection Act to keep personal and sensitive information confidential. The Data Protection Act gives people the right to access information held about them except in certain situations. Representatives acting on behalf of the person, who are deemed competent to manage their affairs, can see and discuss information held about the individual provided the person has given their consent. Independent

Mental Health Advocates and Independent Mental Capacity Advocates also have the right to access the person's records to enable them to make decisions in the person's best interests.

The Data Protection Act is not a barrier; it is a framework to ensure that information about a living person is shared correctly. It is important that you are honest and transparent with the person and their family about **why, what, how and with whom** information might be shared.

Some things to consider:

- If in doubt seek advice and be sure you have access to your policies on confidentiality and record sharing at work.
- Ensure that any record keeping is objective and clear to whoever reads it. All records should be dated and contain the name of the person who has written the record.
- Share records with consent when possible, and try to respect the wishes of the person with dementia.
- You may need to share information with carers and others without consent, if, in the judgement of your manager and/or organisation, that lack of consent can be overridden in the interest of the person or the public. You must also base these decisions on the safety and wellbeing of the person.

If you do share information it must be:

- Necessary: information should be shared on a 'need to know' basis. Do not share anything that is not relevant to the situation.

- Relevant: information shared must only relate to the specific request.
- Accurate: ensure that the information is a true and objective reflection of the person or circumstances. It should not include opinions.
- Timely: be prompt in sharing the information and make sure it is dated and up to date.
- Secure: information should be stored and transported as safely as possible.

LO2 Be able to maximise the rights and choices of individuals with dementia

2.1 **Demonstrate that the best interests of an individual with dementia are considered when planning and delivering care and support**

We have learnt that the 'best interests' of a person with dementia are protected by the Mental Capacity Act. In order to maximise the rights and choices of the person we must always presume they have capacity unless we can show evidence that indicates otherwise.

There may also be occasions when the person with dementia is in hospital for medical treatment and decisions need to be made about their future care. Being in hospital (or any strange environment) can also affect the ability of the person. It might be in their best interests to wait until their medical treatment has finished before expecting them to make an insightful decision. People with dementia can be easily influenced and as vulnerable adults must be protected from being persuaded to make decisions when they may not be able to exercise their full capacity.

We should always encourage the person to participate in the planning of their care and support.

If this is difficult because of the impact of their dementia, consider their past wishes and preferences. Are there any **Advanced Wishes (Living Wills)**?

Case Study

 1.3 Mrs Jones

Mrs Jones lives alone and receives care at home. She is beginning to show signs of forgetfulness and has been known to go to her neighbour's house in the middle of the night. The neighbour is getting very anxious and has been talking to the social worker. She asks her to tell her about Mrs Jones' diagnosis and what the social worker is going to do as it seems to her Mrs Jones should be in a home. She asks to see the social workers assessment as she feels she has the right as Mrs Jones' neighbour.

What do you think the correct response of the social worker should be?

Key terms

Advanced Wishes are decisions made by the person before losing the capacity to do so.

Think about their values and preferences that would be likely to influence their choices if they had capacity. Talk to family and friends about what their wishes and preferences were before they were unable to make an informed decision. Act in the best interest of the person, not their family or friends.

Do not make assumptions about best interests based on age, gender or behaviour.

 Case Study

 Mrs Jones

Mrs Jones is now admitted to your care home. She has had a mental capacity assessment and the 'best interest' assessor has asked for a particular care plan to be put in place. From her assessment you know that Mrs Jones used to be a seamstress and that she liked to attend church every week. Before she was ill she used to tell her neighbour that 'whatever happens I must have my hair done every week and I need to go to church'. Mrs Jones is now unable to cope with going to church.

What would her care plan include in considering her best interests?

2.2 Demonstrate how an individual with dementia can be enabled to exercise their rights and choices even when a decision has not been deemed to be in their best interests

We can define 'best interest' as supporting the financial, health, emotional and social wellbeing of an individual and taking into consideration their past and present wishes and feelings, advance directives, beliefs and values.

A decision should not be taken if it is not in the person's best interests. There can be a conflict of opinion when the person with dementia lacks the capacity to make specific decisions. A family member may, for example, feel that their relative should go into a care home permanently, whilst the assessor may think that this may only need to be a temporary measure. This could be because it has been assessed as not in the best interest of the person to give up their home without a further period of assessment and recovery. In these situations it is important that the person with dementia is enabled to exercise rights and choices. The assessor would use measures in the Mental Capacity Act to determine how much capacity the person had to make informed decisions about each aspect of the process. Using this and any advanced directives or wishes, they can weigh up what is in the best interest of the person.

Evidence activity

 Give an example of a situation where you have come across a disagreement about decisions for care arrangements. What was the role of the professional staff in this scenario? What did they do to resolve the situation – how did they ensure the rights and choices of the person were acknowledged and respected?

2.3 Explain why it is important not to assume that an individual with dementia cannot make their own decisions

It could be very easy to discriminate against a person with dementia by assuming that:

Dementia = lack of capacity (to make any decision)

It is still common to hear the phrase 'they do not have capacity'. However, we all have capacity in varying degrees, depending on our knowledge, mental health and the type of decision that is to be made. 'Lacking capacity' is a sweeping statement that suggests that a person with dementia automatically has to give up any right to choice and decision-making. This is not the case and it is up to us to empower the person.

Time to reflect

 2.3 **Personal decisions**

Reflect on the different decisions you make every day. They will vary from 'routine' ones like choosing what to wear, to bigger decisions like 'should I apply for a new job'? Consider the person with dementia. Even if they lack capacity to make some of the more complex and difficult decisions like how to manage their finances, they have the right to exercise choice, self-determination and decision-making and should be encouraged to do so. What kind of day-to-day decisions could the person be making and how can you enable and support them to do so?

LO3 Be able to involve carers and others in supporting individuals with dementia

'Others' includes: care workers, social workers, GPs, health workers, IMCAs and IMHAs and support groups.

2.4 **Describe how the ability of an individual with dementia to make decisions may fluctuate**

There will be times when a person may have fluctuating (changing) capacity, for example when they are unwell. Think about a time when you were ill. It is likely that you found it more difficult to make decisions. If a person with dementia has an infection, for example, and has a delirium, it would be unfair to expect them to make informed choices at that point. It is good practice and working in **their best interests** to wait until they are better.

It is not only physical ill health that can affect decision making skills; mental ill health can also have an impact. If the person is depressed they may find it more difficult to think things through and lack the confidence to make decisions.

There are other external factors that can influence the ability of the person to make decisions. People with dementia can have great difficulty adjusting to change – they can become more disoriented and confused and decision making is more difficult.

Under- or over-stimulation may also affect the person. Too much noise, people speaking at once etc. can overwhelm the person and stop them from understanding the decision making process. Under-stimulation, when the person is not engaged in conversations and interactions, lessens their ability to communicate their decisions and to use thought processes.

3.1 **Demonstrate how carers and others can be involved in planning support that promotes the rights and choices of an individual with dementia and minimises risk of harm**

Personalised care planning ensures that the person's rights to make or influence decisions are respected. There will be situations when the person with dementia does not have the capacity to plan their support and their carers and other people who may be supporting them in a professional capacity will be required to plan their care.

It is still vital to place the needs, wishes and preferences of the person at the heart of this process. Carers and others must take into account any advanced wishes of the person and if necessary an independent advocate should offer support. Anyone who is acting on behalf of the person should do so in a legally authorised way, or because the person with dementia agreed to it before they lacked capacity, or because the person supporting them has powers under a **Lasting Power of Attorney**.

Key terms

A Lasting Power of Attorney (LPA) is a legal document that allows you to appoint someone to make decisions about your welfare, money or property. It can be used at any time when you are not able to make your own decisions. There are two types of LPA, one which gives the appointed person the authority to manage your financial affairs and another which also authorises the person to make decisions about your future care arrangements. LPAs are monitored by the Court of Protection.

Being 'next of kin' does not necessarily give you an automatic right to plan the support of a relative with dementia. In order to promote rights and choices and minimise risks, it must be assessed that the carer is acting in the person's best interests.

Evidence activity

(3.1) Promoting and protecting interests

Find out about the Court of Protection and how it can protect the interests of a person with dementia. Talk to colleagues or managers about how they and others have had to support a carer to plan the services for a person with dementia. What were the main issues in protecting the person from harm and promoting their rights?

(3.2) Describe how a conflict of interest can be addressed between the carer and an individual with dementia whilst balancing rights, choices and risk

When we talk about a conflict of interest we mean that the carer may have one opinion about the care needs and future of the person with dementia and the person may have a very different view. Sometimes this is because the person with dementia has limited insight into their situation and is unaware of the risks. Equally, it can also be the case that the carer is 'risk averse', that they are worried about the safety of their relative and do not want them to have a degree of independence. The role of others in such situations is to ensure that the correct assessments of need and risk have been completed to provide as much evidence and support as possible. They should be open about this and engage with the person with dementia and their carer as much as possible, by involving them in the assessments and problem solving. People should be given the information they need to make choices and understand the risks and benefits of the options open to them.

Once comprehensive assessments have been made it may be possible to negotiate some practical solutions which will both ensure the person's rights and choices are upheld whilst minimising risk. It should be remembered that it is rarely possible to eliminate risk completely, but we can put in 'protective measures' to reduce risk. Positive risk taking is beneficial.

Evidence activity

(3.2) Taking risks

Think about the risks you take each day. Make a table of what you think are the positive risks and those you could have avoided. How would you feel if you were told you could not take some of these risks?

There are some situations when the person with dementia is being deprived of their liberty in a care home or hospital and the person is unhappy with this arrangement but the family are concerned that their relative might leave the care home and put themselves at risk.

A best interests assessor may be required to assess the situation, and having taken all views, reports assessments and care planning into consideration will make recommendations in the best interests of the person. They may recommend, for example, that the person should remain in a care home, but with certain adjustments to the care plan to ensure rights and choices are respected.

Evidence activity

(3.2) Respecting wishes

Describe a situation when a family/carer has not agreed with the person's wishes. What policies and legislation were considered and how was the situation resolved?

(3.3) Describe how to ensure an individual with dementia, carers and others feel able to complain without fear of retribution

The Care Quality Commission guidance says that

'people who use services, or others acting on their behalf, are given encouragement, support and opportunities to raise specific needs or to express concerns relating to equality, diversity and human rights.'

CQC Essential standards of Quality and Safety, page 47.

In their regulations, CQC say that all services must have a complaints system, for identifying, handling and responding to complaints. The service and its registered manager must bring the complaints system to the attention of the service user or the responsible person acting on their behalf. The person making the complaint must be offered support to do so if they require it and any complaint must be fully investigated. A timely response must be made and an action plan drawn up to resolve the problem. These guidelines are intended to ensure that people making a complaint will not be discriminated against.

Complaints procedures should:

- be written in plain English so that they are not full of jargon but easily understood
- be available to all service users, their carers, family and friends
- offer advice and advocacy as necessary, particularly when the person is vulnerable and has no one to act on their behalf

- explain what is required to resolve the complaint with likely time frames
- have thorough investigations
- be investigated by staff who are competent to do so and when possible by someone who was not involved in the circumstances leading up to the complaint.

The most important thing to remember is that an organisation that takes complaints seriously and treats the person who has complained with respect is an organisation that has an open culture. This means that both staff and service users are well supported and that discussion is encouraged and mistakes learnt from rather than hidden. This can be achieved through good staff supervision and 'reflective practice'. It also means that service users are seen as partners or equals who have the right to be consulted and offered choices.

Key terms

Reflective practice helps care workers to look at the way they have supported a person in a certain situation. They can take time to think about how they approached the situation and if there are things they would change or improve.

Research and investigate

(3.3) Complaints procedure

Look at your place of work. How much information is there about complaints? Ask permission to talk to some service users to find out if they are aware of the complaints procedure. Look for a complaints leaflet or something similar. What do you know about the complaints procedure? How could you improve your knowledge and that of your service users?

LO4 Be able to maintain the privacy, dignity and respect of individuals with dementia whilst promoting rights and choices

 Describe how to maintain privacy and dignity when providing personal support for intimate care to an individual with dementia

A person with dementia may need support with washing and dressing, bathing or going to the toilet. These are very personal activities and can cause great distress if not approached properly. It may seem obvious to you that the person is unable to manage their personal care, but remember how they might perceive the world. Supporting with personal care must be person centred and not task orientated. This is not a job to get finished, but rather an interaction with another human being.

Consider how it must feel for the person with dementia. You may see the risks in not helping them to maintain their personal hygiene, but they may think they have already washed because their impaired memory tells them so. Imagine how it must feel to have an apparent stranger (they have forgotten you were in the room five minutes ago) try to remove your clothing or tell you they are taking you to the toilet.

In order to maintain a therapeutic relationship with the person and to maintain their privacy and dignity we must respect the place they are in. Think about what you need to support them with. If they decline or are upset, will it wait until later? Can you distract the person with their favourite song or can you ask a colleague if they will help instead – as your face might not 'fit'. Keep looking at the situation from the person's point of view. They may need reminding who you are and be reassured that you are there to help but do not give the impression that you are taking over. Try to go at their pace and if they make choices, respect that. The cardigan may not match the skirt or the man may refuse support with shaving. Ask yourself if there is another way to help. Talk to family and friends. Complaints often happen because families are concerned if their relative is not receiving the personal care they need.

Case Study

4.1 Mrs Jones

Mrs Jones has been in the care home for several months and is now having difficulty with her personal care tasks. She cries and nips staff when they attempt to help her wash and dress. Write a person centred care plan for her, bearing in mind she prefers to get up later, likes to sing her favourite hymns and is very fond of two particular care staff. What would be your contingency plan be if Mrs Jones continues to resist help with personal care. Who could help you? How would you ensure you were working in her best interests?

4.2 Demonstrate that key physical aspects of the environment are enabling care workers to show respect and dignity for an individual with dementia

We have talked about the social model of disability and how the environment can disable the person with dementia. In order to show respect and maintain the dignity of people with dementia the physical environment must be sympathetic to their needs. There are many elements of the environment which should be considered as both supporting dignity and minimising risk. Environments should also be enriching places.

Signage: Signs are only effective if they are meaningful to the person with dementia. Words like 'dining room' or 'toilet' should be accompanied by the correct symbols. Rather than try to make home-made signs it is preferable to take specialist advice. We cannot assume that the person will see the signs, particularly if they have visual impairment. Therefore, do not rely completely on signage. To do so disadvantages the person.

Colour: People with dementia have difficulty with perceptual awareness and an environment with too many patterns and colours can be very confusing. Circles on carpets can be seen as holes to avoid and lines as thresholds to be stepped over. Colour contrasts are very helpful. Contrasting door handles in primary colours and bright toilet seats are helpful as they help the person to differentiate and judge distances.

Furniture: Chairs should be a contrasting colour to the floor. There should not be too much clutter so that the person with dementia is not presented with an obstacle course.

Technology: Assistive technology can be very supportive, particularly for people living in their own homes. Flood, gas and heat detectors can minimise risk. Bed and door sensors are helpful in care homes because they can alert staff to a person moving about without having to constantly invade their privacy.

Room layout: It is important that a room layout is not moved about so the person can become familiar with it. It is helpful in en suite bedrooms if the toilet is in sight from the bed. Care should be taken with mirrors, pictures and windows, because reflections and shadows can be misperceived.

Storage, space for personal belongings: Respect must be shown for the person's belongings by ensuring they have locked facilities and that staff do not move treasured items. If you are visiting the person in their own home bear in mind that you are a guest in their home and as such must respect their space.

Evidence activity

 Enhancing respect and dignity through the environment

Choose one aspect of an environment that you work in, for example signage or furniture. Discuss the potential issues for the person with dementia with your colleagues. How could you enhance the dignity of the person with dementia?

 4.3 **Demonstrate that key social aspects of the environment are enabling care workers to show respect and dignity for an individual with dementia**

It is not only the physical aspects of an environment that can have a positive effect on people with dementia, the way we interact is also crucial. Tom Kitwood used the phrase 'malignant social psychology' which describes how our negative behaviour ignores respect and dignity for the person with dementia. Key social aspects include communication skills (see Chapter 3).

As care workers we must always respect the right of the person to expect a professional approach from us. This means that we should be aware of our own professional boundaries. We may be friendly and supportive but not be 'friends' with the person. This is to prevent a conflict of interest, loss of confidentiality and to protect the person from potential abuse. We must try to remain objective so that we can assess the person and support them in the most effective way.

Team work is also important. We are not able to exclusively support the person, and so the team must work together in a connected way. The person with dementia needs a consistency of approach.

Evidence activity

4.3 **Dos and don'ts**

Compile a list of the dos and don'ts of how you should adopt a professional approach when working with a person with dementia.

Useful website addresses and resources

www.legislation.gov.uk
www.alzheimers.org.uk
www.direct.gov.uk
www.mind.org.uk
www.cqc.org.uk

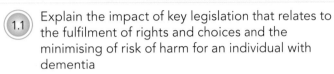

Assessment Summary DEM 304

Reading this unit and completing the activities will have provided you with knowledge, understanding and skills required to promote individuals' rights and choices whilst minimising risk.

To achieve the unit, your assessor will require you to:

Learning Outcomes	Assessment Criteria
1 Understand key legislation and agreed ways of working that support the fulfilment of rights and choices of individuals with dementia while minimising risk of harm	Explain the impact of key legislation that relates to the fulfilment of rights and choices and the minimising of risk of harm for an individual with dementia See research and investigate activity 1.1, page 162
	Evaluate agreed ways of working that relate to the rights and choices of an individual with dementia See evidence activity 1.2, page 163
	Explain how and when personal information may be shared with carers and others, taking into account legislative frameworks and agreed ways of working See case study 1.3, page 164
2 Be able to maximise the rights and choices of individuals with dementia	**2.1** Demonstrate that the best interests of an individual with dementia are considered when planning and delivering care and support See case study 2.1, page 165
	2.2 Demonstrate how an individual with dementia can be enabled to exercise their rights and choices even when a decision has not been deemed to be in their best interests. See evidence activity 2.2, page 165
	2.3 Explain why it is important not to assume that an individual with dementia cannot make their own decisions See time to reflect 2.3, page 165
	2.4 Describe how the ability of an individual with dementia to make decisions may fluctuate See evidence activity 2.4, page 166

Learning Outcomes	Assessment Criteria
3 Be able to involve carers and others in supporting individuals with dementia	**(3.1)** Demonstrate how carers and others can be involved in planning support that promotes the rights and choices of an individual with dementia and minimises risk of harm See evidence activity 3.1, page 166
	(3.2) Describe how a conflict of interest can be addressed between the carer and an individual with dementia whilst balancing rights, choices and risk See evidence activities 3.2, page 167
	(3.3) Describe how to ensure an individual with dementia, carers and others feel able to complain without fear of retribution See research and investigate 3.3, page 168
4 Be able to maintain the privacy, dignity and respect of individuals with dementia whilst promoting rights and choices	**(4.1)** Describe how to maintain privacy and dignity when providing personal support for intimate care to an individual with dementia See case study 4.1, page 168
	(4.2) Demonstrate that key physical aspects of the environment are enabling care workers to show respect and dignity for an individual with dementia See evidence activity 4.2, page 169
	(4.3) Demonstrate that key social aspects of the environment are enabling care workers to show respect and dignity for an individual with dementia See evidence activity 4.3, page 170

Nutritional Needs in Dementia

DEM 302 Understand and meet the nutritional requirements of individuals with dementia

What are you finding out?

Dementia is a condition that is characterised by the progressive decline of brain function and the ability to go about everyday tasks. One of the key tasks that we do everyday often without thinking about it is eating and drinking. This unit is about understanding that individuals may have specific nutritional needs because of their experience of dementia. It is very important that individuals with dementia have their needs and preferences recognised and understood.

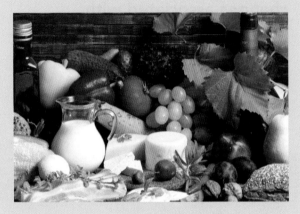

Figure 6.1

Reading this unit and completing the activities will allow you to:

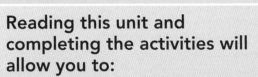

- Understand the nutritional needs that are unique to individuals with dementia

- Understand the effect that mealtime environments can have on an individual with dementia

- Be able to support an individual with dementia to enjoy good nutrition

Key terms

Person centred approach this is a way of working which aims to put the person at the centre of the care situation taking into account their individuality, wishes and preferences.

LO1 Understand the nutritional needs that are unique to individuals with dementia

1.1 Describe how cognitive, functional and emotional changes associated with dementia can affect eating, drinking and nutrition

As a support worker you can provide a range of food and drink in a variety of ways to individuals who use or live within your workplace. In addition to thinking about how nutrition and hydration may be different for people who come from **diverse** backgrounds it is also crucial to consider the changing needs of individuals with dementia as they move through the **dementia journey**. These can be cognitive, physical or functional and emotional changes. These can also present as combinations.

Key terms

Diversity means that people come from a variety of backgrounds.

Dementia journey is the process of moving through the progressive stages of dementia.

Cognitive
- loss of sensory skills, taste, smell, touch
- may eat with hands
- difficulty in communicating hunger and thirst
- inability to chew.

Physical or functional
- swallowing
- loss of sense of smell
- dental or oral problems
- prefer sweet food.

Emotional
- embarrassment
- forget to eat
- forgotten they have eaten
- find it difficult to make a choice
- be suspicious or paranoid
- refuse to eat.

It is also important to consider that due to the progressive nature of dementia **appetite** maybe suppressed or overactive due to lesions in the brain that manage areas responsible for telling us that we are hungry or thirsty. This is because the messages that are sent from the digestive system to the **endocrine systems** are not functioning the way the way they used to due to areas of the brain being affected. Furthermore, it is also important to understand that medication may also affect the appetite and willingness to eat and drink.

Key terms

Appetite is the natural urge that compels us to eat and drink to satisfy body needs.

Endocrine systems are responsible for the production of various hormones and chemical messages that command the physical body to eat, drink, sleep, sexual needs and other fundamental human functions.

The process of eating and drinking is not only to meet the physical needs it plays an important role in how individuals with dementia feel socially and emotionally.

Evidence activity

1.1 How dementia affects nutrition

You have noticed that Mr Smith has been losing weight over the last two weeks. He has started to eat with his hands and says he has not had his breakfast and gets upset when he sees other people eating. He has recently started new medication for a small infection in his mouth but thinks the tablets are to poison him. List the changes that you think Mr Smith maybe experiencing.

1.2 Explain how poor nutrition can contribute to an individual's experience of dementia

There are a number of concerns that are related to poor nutrition and hydration that can contribute negatively to the experiences of people with a diagnosis of dementia. The main areas of concern are:

- lack of calorific intake for day-to-day energy consumption
- lack of protein
- reduced access to and intake of vitamins
- dehydration.

Table 6.1 Effects of poor nutrition

Physical
Risk of infection
Reduces wound healing
Dermatological problems
Constipation
Disturbed sleeping patterns
Weight loss/gain
Reduced brain function
Anaemia

Social and psychological effects
Apathy
Confusion
Memory loss
Delirium
Disturbed sleeping patterns
Mood

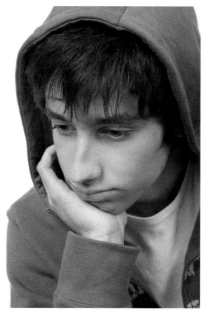

Figure 6.2 Apathy

Evidence activity

1.2 Effects of poor nutrition

1. How do you feel when you have not had anything to eat? Think about your mood, pain and energy levels and make a list.
2. Using the list you have created, then list how these may affect an individual with dementia.
3. Think about the physical and social effects. How do you think the lists combined could affect an individual with dementia?

Key terms

Apathy is a general lack of interest in everyday activities.

1.3 Outline how other health and emotional conditions may affect the nutritional needs of an individual with dementia

As we grow older our bodies change. There are changes, for example, in flexibility, muscle tone, bone thickness, endocrine systems and the amounts of energy that our bodies use. Older people also tend to experience more episodes of ill health. Therefore it is important to maintain a healthy balanced diet to ensure good nutrition and hydration. Older people with dementia tend to be more at risk of poor nutrition and hydration for a number of reasons.

As we get older we do not move around quite so much. The less we move the less calorific intake we obviously require, and therefore people naturally will eat less. However, if the amount of food that an individual with dementia eats does not provide enough nutrition then this can be harmful to the body. If we do not eat enough our bodies do not have access to proteins, carbohydrates, fats and sugars and we then become susceptible to a variety of further risks. Muscles can waste, bones can become brittle and weak. General feelings of weakness and/or limited mobility can diminish confidence in walking, moving around, picking up objects, communicating and coordination.

As well as physical symptoms food also plays a significant role in brain function, mood and the ability to function cognitively. Food and drink contain vitamins and minerals, which are vital to the parts of the brain that send messages, the ways in which the brain reacts and the wider nervous system. Nutrition and hydration are also important in affecting how the body stores good and bad substances around the body. For example, fatty deposits may accumulate in the arteries and veins and may cause heart disease or block arteries. Conditions such as these can cause secondary conditions, such as pressure sores, poor circulation, fluid retention and of course affect mood and willingness to participate on a social level. On the other hand, a lack of iron and protein can cause anaemia. Depression is also a common condition often associated with dementia. Depression can be caused through an awareness of changes in the body and diminishing capabilities and capacities.

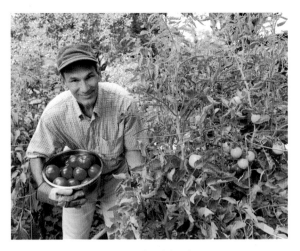
Figure 6.3 Maintaining a healthy diet

Evidence activity

1.3 Emotional and health conditions

This activity will assist your understanding of how physical health conditions can be related to emotional conditions (see 1.1).

List three physical health conditions

1.

2.

3.

List three emotional conditions

1.

2.

3.

1.4 Explain the importance of recognising and meeting an individual's personal and cultural preferences for food and drink

People may have different views and attitudes about foods dependent upon their cultural background. We described this as diversity. Diversity is an important area to consider when thinking about what food and drink people like but also the ways in which they may be accustomed to eating and drinking and with what utensils. It is important to recognise an individual's personal and cultural preference to food and drink as this can make people feel like they are respected and included. This encourages people to eat and drink but can also increase their emotional and physical wellbeing because they are socially included.

In providing a range of food and drink we can also set a scene of familiarity and variety. This can help make individuals feel at home, safe and secure, and a welcome and valued person. A choice of menu can also provide the scope for ensuring good nutrition and hydration.

Cultural backgrounds often mean that different foods mean different things to different people. As well as providing nutritional value food and drink also play a significant role in culture and rituals. For example, Hindus sit on the floor and Chinese people eat with chopsticks. Some people may like to have a glass of wine with their meal and listen to music. Traditional meal time cultures are the ways in which people from different cultural backgrounds like to eat their food. It is important to be aware of diversity and how people from different cultures can only eat certain things, their rituals and ceremonies. It is also important to consider the different times individuals like to eat; this information can be obtained with the life history.

Individuals with dementia will present varying symptoms which may fluctuate throughout the dementia journey. A variety of food and drink can ensure the stages and fluctuations are monitored in a controlled way.

Evidence activity

 1.4 **Cultural preferences**

Think about the different people that you have met recently. What were their cultural backgrounds? Consider the different food and drink that they may eat and drink. Make a list of the different food they eat and how they eat it.

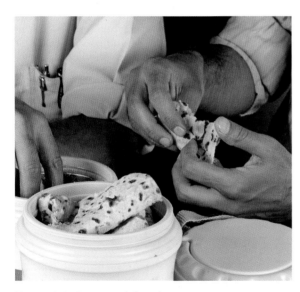

Figure 6.4 Eating with hands

1.5 **Explain why it is important to include a variety of food and drink in the diet of an individual with dementia**

It is important to include a variety of food and drink in the diet of an individual with dementia for a variety of reasons:

- **Nutrition and hydration** – we need a variety of vitamins, minerals and fibre to maintain physical wellbeing.
- **Interest and capabilties** – a balanced diet and variety of meals prevents boredom with food. It is important to make food look appetising. Sometimes food needs to be of different textures for people with swallowing difficulties but it is important to remember that not all food for people with swallowing difficulties needs to be puréed.
- **The quality of the eating experience** – can also be improved by offering a variety of foods. If you do think that food and drink intake is proving to be a problem then advice can be obtained from a speech and language therapist. The table layout and room can also contribute positively.

Evidence activity

1.5 **The importance of variety**

Explain why it is important to include a variety of food and drink in the diet of an individual with dementia.

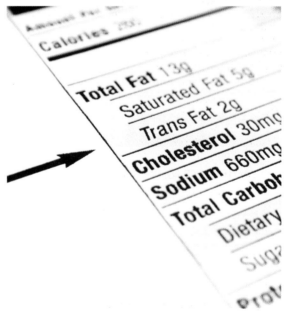

Figure 6.5 Nutrition information

LO2 Understand the effect that mealtime environments can have on an individual with dementia

Describe how mealtime cultures and environments can be a barrier to meeting the nutritional needs of an individual with dementia

Research has shown that mealtime cultures and environments can be a barrier to meeting the nutritional needs of an individual with dementia. The ways in which we do things or perform tasks can be described as a culture. The way a room is set out can be described as the physical environment. Barriers can include both the physical and social environment. For example, a dining room which is not sensitive to the needs of individuals with dementia can hinder food and drink intake and cause a negative social atmosphere. Issues such as staff talking over one another can create a negative element to the dining experience. The mealtime cultures and environments can hinder interactions which create stimulation and enjoyment through:

- lack of opportunities to socialise
- reduced abilities to engage with familiar activities
- lack of access to activities such as reminiscence, listening to favourite music, baking
- restricted social routines, such as going to the fish and chip shop, out for coffee and so on.

Evidence activity

(2.1) Barriers at mealtime

What do you think would cause barriers to the nutrition and hydration of individuals with dementia with the mealtime cultures and environments in your work setting?

Describe how mealtime environments and food presentation can be designed to help an individual to eat and drink

Mealtime environments are crucial to how individuals with dementia and their carers experience eating and drinking. This can mean the difference between enjoying it or finding the experience unpleasant and food and drink intake being inadequate. In this section we will consider the design of the environment and discuss how design can help or place significant barriers to an individual's ability to perform this important everyday task. It is useful to think of the environment in two ways.

The physical environment

The physical environment has a significant impact on individuals' ability to eat and drink independently. For example, the way in which the table is set, the room is set out and even the corridor leading up to the dining room can assist in providing an enabling environment. As we grow older our bodies change due to the natural ageing process. Our eyesight can deteriorate and hearing can become impaired. Our ability to move or pick things up can also be affected through conditions such as arthritis or rheumatism. These are all symptomatic of conditions synonymous with the natural ageing process. Therefore it is very important to put careful consideration into how you design the dining area and present your food and drink. It is helpful to think of the experience as a journey. We shall now consider the journey to the dining room area.

Evidence activity

(2.2) The physical environment

Think about the journey or route to the dining room in your workplace and any improvements that could be made to aid the individual with dementia.

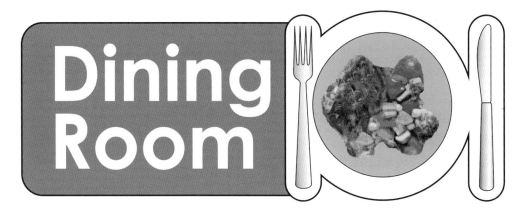

Figure 6.6 Clear signage

The corridor

The corridor leading into the dining room can be improved by putting a few pictures of food on the walls at a height that can be seen. These pictures can begin to stimulate appetite and assist on orientation and way-finding. The door should be situated so that tables and chairs can be easily seen.

The dining room

The doorway of the dining room should present a sign that denotes the dining room area. Signage designed specifically for people with a range of cognitive and physical impairments tend to use the multiple cue concept. These should include photos or realistic pictures representing the areas that you are signing. The font should use capital letters first followed by lower case. It should use bright colours that stand out from the background and a matt laminate.

Again, pictures of food on the walls can assist with orientation and also stimulate the appetite of the residents. The room should be quiet and mealtimes should be protected. Phone calls should not be made or taken unless it is an emergency and once a resident has started eating then they should not be moved until they have finished.

The manner in which the table is set can aid enormously with enhancing the eating and drinking experience. The traditional manner in which a dining table is set tends to use white table cloths, white crockery and clear glass. People who have visual impairments find it difficult to distinguish contrast between surfaces. In Chapter 1 we discussed how individuals with dementia or dementia syndrome may present or experience symptoms such as delusions, difficulty in communicating, coordination, movement and spatial awareness that can exacerbate natural symptoms of ageing. White table cloths and white crockery can make it difficult for individuals with dementia to recognise there is a plate or dish on the table. This can be made even more problematic if a pale food such as mash potato or rice pudding is offered for a meal. Clear glasses containing water are also difficult to see and may be ignored or knocked over. Knives and forks can be difficult to use and getting food onto cutlery and into the mouth can be difficult and present significant

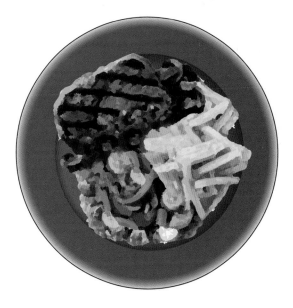

Figure 6.7 Coloured plates can make food easier to see

problems for individuals with dementia. These types of difficulties and problems can lead to losing confidence, feelings of embarrassment, malnutrition and dehydration, loss of skill sets and social withdrawal. Other factors to be taken into consideration are whether the individual's dentures fit and whether they have recently been to the toilet.

Evidence activity

 2.2 Designing a mealtime environment

What elements of your dining room could be improved to help an individual with dementia eat and drink?

Case Study

 2.2 Ella

Ella has been getting increasingly upset at meal times. It seems as soon as her support worker goes into the living room to take her in her wheelchair for her lunch she becomes agitated and says she needs the toilet. However, even after she has been taken to the toilet Ella is still upset. Her mood seems to get worse when she is taken into the dining room. Ella used to help others around her but now she gets cross with people sitting next to her and refuses to feed herself. Ella's support worker is concerned that she does not eat or drink in the dining room any more as she used to be an independent woman who liked to help others around her.

Ella seems to be happier to eat sandwiches, cold meat and cake in her room.

What action could Ella's support worker take to understand better the situation?

What areas do you think could be problematic for Ella?

Social environment

The art of eating and drinking is not just a physical necessity but a social activity. Eating and drinking in the dining room is an important time where residents will get the opportunity to interact with fellow residents, staff and families. The ways in which people behave and the manner in which we behave towards others is affected by the social environment we create around us. The social environment is based on social **interactions** with people and the physical environment. It is important that support workers notice these behaviours and physiological symptoms.

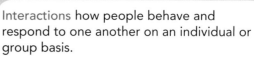 **Key terms**

Interactions how people behave and respond to one another on an individual or group basis.

 2.3 Describe how a person centred approach can support an individual, with dementia at different levels of ability, to eat and drink

Exercising a person centred approach and incorporating this into your work attitude is useful on many levels. By being person centred you take time to listen and ask questions so that you can learn about what individuals like and dislike. Being person centred also allows you to be able to think and prepare when assisting people with what they like or prefer. Being person centred can improve an individual's sense of wellbeing.

Setting the scene

In considering a person centred approach to food setting the scene is important. Make food an activity – thinking about making mealtimes as an activity can promote interest and improve mood. For example, think about traditions. Fish is traditionally eaten on Fridays. Therefore fish and chips eaten from the fish and chip shop can provide a variety of opportunities for activities such as learning what each individual likes to buy from the fish and chip shop and a supervised outing to the local fish and chip shop. If this is not possible then this activity may still be carried out by placing fish and chips cooked within your work environment and placed on appropriate paper, just as you may find at a fish and chip shop. This type of activity can be replicated with any traditions.

A person centred approach also considers the language used around food. For example, teacake, barm, bread roll and baps all mean the same thing but are used in different dialects.

Evidence activity

Evidence activity

 Providing a person centred experience

Think about the different cultures, seasonal and family traditions that could provide a list of traditions to help you make nutrition into an activity.

	Day	Season	Event	Family
Tradition				
Activity				

LO3 Be able to support an individual with dementia to enjoy good nutrition

In this section we will consider how to provide support for individuals to enjoy good nutrition.

3.1 Demonstrate how the knowledge of life history of an individual with dementia has been used to provide a diet that meets his/her preferences

Life history work aims to gather and collate information about individuals. Life history work is useful because it gives us important knowledge about what a person's preferences are and the ways in which they like to do things. It can consist of autobiographical work, personal narratives, such as talking, storytelling and memorabilia. See **www.lifestorynetwork.org.uk** for further details. Life history work seeks to understand what preferences individuals have by taking their perspectives into consideration. Life history tools allow us to understand the times people may prefer to eat, the foods they like or dislike, whether they like listening to music and so on. It can also provide insights into the good and bad experiences that may be associated with mealtimes, and provides opportunities to understand what foods individuals may prefer or have for special occasions.

Evidence activity

 Using life history

Develop a life story tool that considers feelings as well as facts. What do they find interesting? What foods do they like when they are hot or cold, feel sad, want comfort food? How do they take their tea or coffee? What are their food preferences?

3.2 Demonstrate how mealtimes for an individual with dementia are planned to support his/her ability to eat and drink

As we have learned through this chapter, nutrition and hydration is crucial for the physical wellbeing of individuals with dementia. Food and drink is also about emotional and social wellbeing and is an area of our lives where we make lots of decisions. It is important to get to know people, their preferences and keep up to date records on their abilities and capabilities in order to support them to eat and drink.

3.3 Demonstrate how the specific eating and drinking abilities and needs of an individual with dementia have been addressed

Individuals with dementia may have specific eating and drinking abilities. These are often unique and require detailed records to be kept to monitor the capability to eat and drink. Throughout this unit we have addressed cognitive, functional and emotional changes, the process of natural ageing, diversity and the importance of a varied diet. In addition we have also considered how the physical and social environment can prove to be a barrier for nutrition and hydration, and provided solutions to common problems. We have also considered

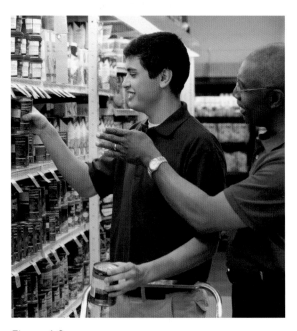

Figure 6.8

tools that are useful for gathering information about individuals that we can use to provide care and support by recognising that each individual with dementia is unique.

3.4 Demonstrate how a person centred approach to meeting nutritional requirements has improved the wellbeing of an individual with dementia

Adopting a person centred approach to meeting nutritional requirements can improve the wellbeing of individuals with dementia by ensuring that they have access to vitamins, minerals and proteins. In addition, embracing a person centred approach also provides excellent opportunities for individual and social activities. Therefore when an individual is consulted about their heritage, culture, preferences and dislikes and are actively participating in mealtime activities then their physical health and wellbeing are being improved. As we have discussed physical needs can be linked with social needs. Therefore by adopting a person centred approach this can also improve mental health due to sense of inclusion, dignity, confidence and overall wellbeing of an individual with dementia. For the purpose of this unit wellbeing is understood to mean:

- appropriate weight gain/loss
- improved sleep patterns
- reduced confusion
- improved physical health
- improved emotional state
- reduced infections
- reduced constipation.

Case Study

 Mrs Cassidy

Mrs Cassidy moved into a care home two years ago and used to enjoy mealtimes. She looked forward to these times as it gave her time with her fellow residents and the food was lovely. When Mrs Cassidy moved into the care home she was in early to moderate stage of her dementia journey. She was still able to feed herself because her skill sets were still intact but over the last year she has found it increasingly difficult to see the food on her plate and becomes confused with the table setting often knocking over glasses of water and dropping her food down her front. This makes Mrs Cassidy feel very embarrassed. The noise in the dining room also makes her feel disorientated and a little anxious. Therefore Mrs Cassidy decides that she does not want to go into the dining room anymore to eat her food. Instead she stays in her room and eats sandwiches because she can manage those with no problems. Mrs Cassidy's support worker had just returned from a training course that highlighted how mealtime experiences could be improved.

Mrs Cassidy, along with all the other residents, was asked about the food they would like to have on the menu. The dining room was fitted with soft furnishings to lower the noise and echoes and table settings were changed using brightly coloured crockery and adapted cutlery. Mrs Cassidy was a very curious lady so asked to go down to lunch just to see what changes had occurred. That day Mrs Cassidy did not have sandwiches for lunch, instead she tried some of the cottage pie and apple crumble. She found it much easier to see the food and was able to feed herself with the new crockery and forks. Mrs Cassidy felt much more comfortable and laughed with her old friend that she had not seen for months. Mrs Cassidy began to go down to the dining room again and her records showed that she had regained a little weight, her mood had improved and that she was sleeping much better. The kitchen staff had noticed less food waste and felt happy that the food they were cooking was now being enjoyed much more.

List the ways the person centred approach assisted with improving the wellbeing of Mrs Cassidy.

Assessment Summary DEM 302

Your reading of this unit and completion of the activities will have prepared you to demonstrate your learning and understanding of the nutritional requirements of individuals with dementia.

To achieve the unit, your assessor will require you to:

Learning Outcomes	Assessment Criteria
1 Understand the nutritional needs that are unique to individuals with dementia	Describe how cognitive, functional and emotional changes associated with dementia can affect eating, drinking and nutrition See evidence activity 1.1, page 174
	Explain how poor nutrition can contribute to an individual's experience of dementia See evidence activity 1.2, page 175
	Outline how other health and emotional conditions may affect the nutritional needs of an individual with dementia See evidence activity 1.3, page 176
	Explain the importance of recognising and meeting an individual's personal and cultural preferences for food and drink See evidence activity 1.4, page 177
	Explain why it is important to include a variety of food and drink in the diet of an individual with dementia See evidence activity 1.5, page 177
2 Understand the effect that that mealtime environments can have on an individual with dementia	Describe how mealtime cultures and environments can be a barrier to meeting the nutritional needs of an individual with dementia See evidence activity 2.1, page 178
	Describe how mealtime environments and food presentation can be designed to help an individual to eat and drink See evidence activities 2.2, pages 178 and 180
	Describe how a person centred approach can support an individual, with dementia at different levels of ability, to eat and drink See evidence activity 2.3, page 181

Learning Outcomes	Assessment Criteria
3 Be able to support an individual with dementia to enjoy good nutrition	Demonstrate how the knowledge of life history of an individual with dementia has been used to provide a diet that meets his/her preferences See evidence activity 3.1, page 181
	Demonstrate how mealtimes for an individual with dementia are planned to support his/her ability to eat and drink See evidence activity 3.2, page 182
	Demonstrate how the specific eating and drinking abilities and needs of an individual with dementia have been addressed See evidence activity 3.3, page 182
	Demonstrate how a person centred approach to meeting nutritional requirements has improved the wellbeing of an individual with dementia See case study 3.4, page 183

7 Medication in Dementia
DEM 305 Understand the administration of medication to individuals with dementia using a person centred approach

What are you finding out?

It is important to understand why and how particular medication is given to people with dementia. Although medication can be very beneficial, it has always to be treated with caution and the benefits have to be weighed against the negative aspects or side effects.

Reading through the unit and completing the activities will enable you to:

• Understand the common medications available to, and appropriate for, individuals with dementia

• Understand how to provide person centred care to individuals with dementia through the appropriate and effective use of medication

LO1 Understand the common medications available to, and appropriate for, individuals with dementia

In this section we will look at four main types of medication used specifically to help people with dementia. It is important to remember that **any** drug given to older people can have an adverse effect and the rule that is usually applied to anti-psychotics, or anti-depressants, for example, is 'start low, go slow' This means that drugs are often 'titrated'.

Key terms

Titration is the gradual increase in drug dosage to a level that provides the best therapeutic effect.

The main types of medication we will look at are:

- anti-dementia drugs
- anti-depressants
- anxiolytics
- anti-psychotics

Drugs have at least two names – a **generic** name, which defines what is in the drug, and a **trade name**, which varies depending upon the company that produced it. For example '**Aricept**' is the trade name and '**donepezil hydrochloride**' is the generic name.

1.1 Outline the most common medications used to treat symptoms of dementia

Anti-dementia drugs

The following drugs can be used **only** in the treatment of Alzheimer's disease, not vascular dementia, unless the person has a diagnosis of 'mixed dementia' – that is, has both vascular dementia and Alzheimer's disease.

The drugs that may be prescribed to help people with Alzheimer's disease are not a cure, but can help with some of the symptoms of the disease. The beneficial effects can last for several years but wear off over time. Because they do not stop the disease progressing in the brain, people can

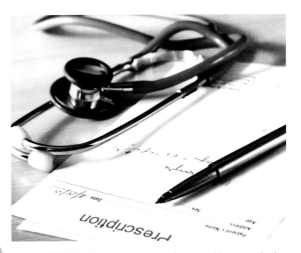

Figure 7.1 It is important to understand how and why medication is prescribed and what its side effects might be.

continue to gradually get worse even though they are taking the medication.

NICE guidelines (2011) acknowledge that the carer as well as the person with dementia should be consulted about the progression of the person's dementia. It recommends that a holistic assessment of the person is made before the medication is prescribed. This means that doctors cannot simply rely on memory tests like the Mini Mental State Examination (MMSE).

Cholinesterase inhibitors

Alzheimer's disease can be treated by two different drug types. The first type are **Cholinesterase inhibitors** and are:

- Aricept (donepezil hydrochloride)
- Reminyl (galantamine)
- Exelon (rivastigmine).

A chemical in the brain called **acetylcholine** acts as a message transmitter and in Alzheimer's disease people lose nerve cells which use this chemical. Aricept, Exelon and Reminyl prevent an enzyme called **acetylcholinesterase** breaking down acetylcholine. An improvement in the production of acetylcholine leads to increased communication between the nerve cells.

The National Institute for Health and Clinical Excellence (NICE) guidelines 2011 recommends that Aricept, Reminyl and Exelon are available as part of NHS care for people with mild-to-moderate Alzheimer's disease. All drugs have to be licensed for a particular use and as yet these drugs are not licensed for use for someone with severe dementia. All these drugs can only be prescribed first by a consultant. The GP can write repeat prescriptions once the medication is assessed to be beneficial to the person with dementia.

Benefits

People with Alzheimer's disease who are treated with one of these drugs can improve in several ways, although it is important to understand that the benefit of this medication is **not long term**. There may be some improvement in:

- activities of daily living skills
- levels of anxiety
- motivation
- memory
- concentration (thinking).

NMDA receptor antagonists

The second type of medicine is an 'NMDA receptor antagonist' called Ebixa (Memantine).

Evidence activity

1.1 Common medications

Think about the ways in which a person's quality of life can improve if they are able to take anti-dementia medication. For example, if they are able to manage some activities of daily living better, how will this impact on their life and that of the carer? What effect could an increased level of motivation have, and so on.

This is the most recent drug. Ebixa blocks a messenger chemical called **glutamate**. Too much glutamate is produced when brain cells are damaged by Alzheimer's disease. Ebixa can protect brain cells by stopping damage from the effects of too much glutamate. It is mainly used in the moderate and severe stages of dementia. It is also helpful in helping with some of the behavioural and psychological symptoms of dementia (BPSD), including aggression.

Side effects (adverse reaction)

People do not react to drugs in the same way. A particular drug may be more successful for some people than others. Equally, not everyone experiences the same side effects. Doctors will

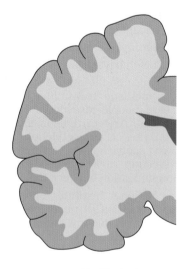
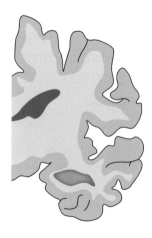

Healthy brain   Servere AD

Figure 7.2 Cholinesterase inhibitors are used in the treatment of Alzheimer's disease.

monitor how a person reacts to a new drug and may have to change the dose or the medication itself if there is an **adverse reaction**.

The most frequent side effects of the cholinesterase inhibitors are:

- loss of appetite
- sickness
- stomach upsets including diarrhoea
- headaches and dizziness
- insomnia.

Time to reflect

1.1 Pros and cons

Think about the reasons a person with Alzheimer's disease may be reluctant to take anti-dementia drugs. What do you think are the pros and cons?

1.2 Describe how commonly used medications affect individuals with dementia

Not everyone with dementia will be prescribed an anti-dementia drug. People with dementia can also feel depressed or anxious or experience hallucinations or periods of agitation. Several types of medication are used to support a person with dementia who may have some of these symptoms.

Anti-depressants

People with dementia can develop depression, which is a mood disorder. Depression has a major impact on people's functioning and quality of life. Mild depression can be treated with psychological treatment called 'talking therapies' and other interventions, but medication is considered in more severe clinical depression.

Depression can have a gradual onset. People who experience depression may have difficulty concentrating, be easily distracted, and have intrusive negative thoughts. They may have feelings of helplessness and low self-esteem. Depression in older people with dementia is common and is easily overlooked or mistaken as a part of the process of dementia. However, it is possible to live well with dementia and so any symptoms of depression must be taken very seriously. People with dementia are one group of people who are more at risk of developing depression. There is still a lot of scientific debate about the usefulness of prescribing anti-depressants for people with dementia and so it is important to look at alternative therapies.

Research and investigate

1.2 Treating depression

What kind of alternative therapies do you think might be helpful for a person who is depressed? We have mentioned talking therapies as one method.

Here are two examples of some of the more common drugs used with older people.

- **Citalopram**. This is a type of anti-depressant called an 'SSRI', or 'Selective Serotonin Re-uptake Inhibitor'. Citalopram helps by rebalancing serotonin levels, as it is thought an imbalance of this chemical can lead to depression. It is considered one of the 'cleaner' anti-depressants as it can result in fewer side effects. Side effects include nausea, dizziness, sleepiness, dry mouth, agitation, confusion.
- **Mirtazapine** works in the brain to increase the amount of noradrenaline and serotonin in order to improve mood and help with depression. Side effects include drowsiness, dizziness, dry mouth, tiredness, shakiness, difficulty sleeping and feelings of hostility.

Anxiolytics

This medication helps in the reduction of symptoms of anxiety and sleeping problems and includes a group of drugs called **benzodiazepines**. They improve the effect of a substance in the brain called GABA which is a neurotransmitter. GABA has a generally calming effect in the human brain.

The main generic drugs in this category are:

- diazepam
- lorazepam
- temazepam
- nitrazepam and
- zopiclone.

Side effects include drowsiness, dizziness, headache, and nausea, unsteadiness and memory loss. These side effects are not always apparent.

1.3 **Explain the risks and benefits of anti-psychotic medication for individuals with dementia**

Anti-psychotics

Psychosis is a condition where the person is unable to differentiate between reality and their imagination. This is evidenced in hallucinations and delusions.

If non-pharmacological interventions have not worked and the person with dementia is exhibiting signs of agitation and distress, the consultant psychiatrist may consider treatment using an anti-psychotic drug. These are also known as **neuroleptics**.

People with dementia can experience behavioural problems such as restlessness or aggression. This is termed 'Behavioural and Psychological Symptoms of Dementia' (BPSD), or psychiatric symptoms such as psychosis (delusions and hallucinations). Anti-psychotics can be used to treat these symptoms, but they have a varying success rate. Most recent evidence shows that there is little value in prescribing an anti-psychotic to a person with dementia unless they have shown physical aggression or have actual psychotic symptoms. It is therefore not recommended for use when a person is wandersome, displays perseveration or is distressed.

Key terms

Perseveration is when a person with dementia continuously repeats a pattern of behaviour or speech. For example, rocking, calling for help.

The British National Formulary (BNF) advises the following:

'Prescribing for the elderly

The balance of risks and benefits should be considered before prescribing anti-psychotic drugs for elderly patients. In elderly patients with dementia anti-psychotic drugs are associated with a small increased risk of mortality and an increased risk of stroke or transient ischaemic attack. …

It is recommended that

- Anti-psychotic drugs should not be used in elderly patients to treat mild to moderate psychotic symptoms
- Treatment should be reviewed regularly '.

Anyone prescribed an anti-psychotic drug should be closely and regularly monitored by a doctor or psychiatric nurse. They should be reviewed within three months.

When the medication is first prescribed it is very important that care staff observe for side effects. They should ensure that the person continues to be mobile and that they drink plenty of fluids. Anti-psychotic medication can make someone drowsy and more reluctant to drink or move about. This in itself will cause medical problems like dehydration and falls.

Some commonly used anti-psychotic drugs include:

- Olanzapine
- Haloperidol and
- Quetiapine.

Many psychotropic drugs have not been trialled in people over the age of 65, and therefore they must be prescribed with caution.

However, one anti-psychotic drug, **Risperidone** is licensed for use in older people with Alzheimer's disease and is therefore the 'drug of choice'. It is recommended for use in the short term for people with moderate to severe dementia who have symptoms of psychosis or are physically aggressive.

Anti-psychotics can have serious side effects. The risk involved in the long-term use of anti-psychotic drugs is associated with an increased risk of stroke and sudden death and may increase cognitive impairment in people with Alzheimer's

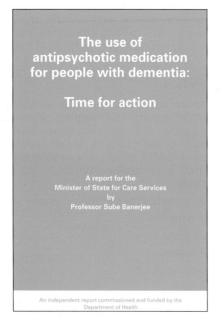

The use of
antipsychotic medication
for people with dementia:

Time for action

A report for the
Minister of State for Care Services
by
Professor Sube Banerjee

An independent report commissioned and funded by the
Department of Health

Figure 7.3 Anti-psychotics should be used with caution and side effects closely monitored.

disease. All anti-psychotics can be very dangerous for people with dementia with Lewy bodies. They can cause symptoms to worsen and, in some cases, sudden death.

In recognition of widespread concern about the over-prescription of anti-psychotic drugs, and as part of the priority being given to improving care for people with dementia, Professor Sube Banerjee was asked to undertake an independent clinical review of the use of anti-psychotic drugs. He argues that too often anti-psychotics are used to treat BPSD rather than a psychosis. He describes BPSD as aggression, wandering, shouting, repeated questions and sleep disturbance and a core syndrome of dementia. It causes distress to both the cared for person and the carer but it is not necessarily a psychosis.

He concludes that:

- anti-psychotics are used too much
- the risks (adverse side effects) outweigh the benefits
- we must reduce the use of anti-psychotics, particularly as a first choice of treatment
- we must use alternative methods to support people with dementia who have BPSD.

He makes recommendations including:

- **Recommendation 6:** The Royal Colleges of General Practitioners, Psychiatrists, Nursing and Physicians should develop a curriculum for the development of appropriate skills for GPs and others working in care homes, to equip them for their role in the management of the complexity, co-morbidity and severity of mental and physical disorder in those now residing in care homes. This should be available as part of continuing professional development.
- **Recommendation 7:** There is a need to develop a curriculum for the development of appropriate skills for care home staff in the non-pharmacological treatment of behavioural disorder in dementia, including the deployment of specific therapies with positive impact. Senior staff in care homes should have these skills and the ability to transfer them to other staff members.

Evidence activity

 Pros and cons of anti-psychotic medication

Write a list of the pros and cons for prescribing anti-psychotic medication.

 Explain the importance of recording and reporting side effects /adverse reactions to medication

This is a direct quote from a carer of a person with dementia who is being supported in a care home. It is taken from Professor Banerjee's report.

'I hold them responsible for his rapid loss of speech, the constant drooling, his mask-like frozen expression, the constant jerking of his right foot that stayed with him for the rest of his life, and rapid onset of incontinence. While still able to walk, he would walk leaning over sideways or backwards at an alarming angle, and no doubt it was this "unbalancing" that caused the hip fractures. Soon he developed epileptic fits and I cannot be sure that it was not related to the anti-psychotics.'

Time to reflect

1.4 Reporting side effects

Think about the comments from this carer. Do you think that the person's side effects were reported in a timely and effective way? How could you have dealt with this situation differently?

Although the doctor will prescribe the medication, it is important that you both report symptoms of the illness and the effect the medication has on those symptoms. We have already learned that we must not assume a person with dementia behaves in a certain way. Any changes (improvements or deterioration) should be communicated to the doctor who can make a re-assessment of the person and therefore make informed decisions about the medication they prescribe. It is always important to establish a 'baseline' which means you have a clear understanding of how the person usually behaves, reacts and so on. You are therefore looking at changes to whatever is 'normal' for them.

The side effects of medication can be very serious, sometimes with devastating consequences. A greater risk of falls or lack of appetite or further deterioration in memory worsens the situation for a person with dementia. If you are aware of the side effects you can, by observing closely and reporting change accurately, ensure that any problems are dealt with as soon as possible.

It is also important to alert the doctor when the person does not comply with their medication. Accurate recording on medication charts is very important because it not only evidences the administration of medication as a legal document; it also highlights any errors or omissions.

People with dementia may have problems complying with medication because they do not understand how to take the medication, or they find it difficult to swallow, or they simply forget to take it. Again, appropriate adjustments can be made if this is recorded and reported in a timely way.

Polypharmacy

Key terms

Polypharmacy is defined as the practice of prescribing four or more medications to the same person (Department of Health, 2001).

Older people with dementia will probably experience other medical conditions like arthritis, diabetes, heart conditions, vascular problems, cancer or digestive problems. These medical problems may also require treatment with certain medication. All medication should therefore be reviewed regularly to confirm whether continued prescribing is necessary.

The risks which contribute to polypharmacy are:

- Repeat prescriptions. Older people living alone or with little support may struggle to manage their medicine management. If their prescriptions are not regularly reviewed it is possible that they continue taking too many different medications.

- Poor communication between support workers or families and the GP. Any changes or concerns should be reported to the GP as soon as possible. They can then review the medication and change, reduce or even stop it as necessary.

- Using guidelines without using a person centred approach. We must always remember 'person first, dementia second'. Think about what is best for the person. Seek their views and those of their family/carer. Medication should not be prescribed in an isolated way, but rather looking at the whole picture, using the evidence of a holistic assessment.

The adverse effects of polypharmacy are primarily premature morbidity and increased risk of falls and delirium (an acute confusional state).

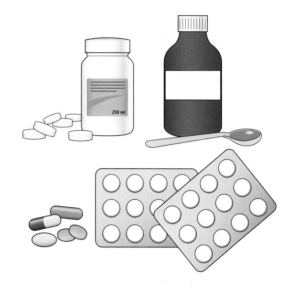

Figure 7.4 More than four prescribed medications is termed polypharmacy and can cause confusion or falls.

1.5 Describe how 'as required' (PRN) medication can be used to support individuals with dementia who may be in pain

A person with dementia feels pain, just like you or me. They can experience painful conditions like arthritis, for example. However, they may not be able to tell you verbally in a way that you will easily understand. We must never assume that someone is **not** in pain just because they do not say so. A person who has poor short-term memory may only 'be' in the moment and therefore can only tell you that they are in pain at the time you ask. They may not remember several minutes later, or the next day, but they could still be experiencing pain.

If a person with dementia is in pain and cannot tell you verbally, it is very important you use your communication skills (see Chapter 3) and look for non-verbal signs.

In fact, some of the ways a person might behave are the kinds of behaviour that we can find the most challenging to support, and we might even dismissed them as 'just part of the dementia'.

Time to reflect

1.5 PRN medication

Think about the behaviour and noises that may indicate a person with dementia is in pain – what are the clues?

In a recent research project in care homes, the researchers wanted to find out whether giving pain control regularly to people with moderate to severe dementia could reduce agitation. They concluded that this agitation was significantly reduced if people were given daily treatment for pain.

Time to reflect

1.5

Think about this research. What does it tell us about agitation and aggression? What significance does this have when we realise that anti-psychotics are often the first line of treatment for agitation?

Although giving pain control 'when necessary' (PRN) may be appropriate for people who can tell you clearly when they are in pain, or are able to explain where the pain is, or how intense it feels, this is not necessarily the case for a person with dementia. If the person has been prescribed regular pain control then it should be given regularly. If you think a person is in pain because you have observed non-verbal signs, or have been able to complete an assessment, it is equally important to seek medical advice as soon as possible.

Types of pain control include:

- Paracetamol
- Morphine and
- Pregabalin. Pregabalin can also be used for the management of anxiety.

Like all medication, painkillers also have side effects and it is important to note these when giving regular pain relief as sometimes they can introduce further problems like constipation.

Research and investigate

1.5 Paracetamol, morphine and pregabaline

Find out more about these three drugs. When are they used, what are the doses and what are their side effects?

LO2 Understand how to provide person centred care to individuals with dementia through the appropriate and effective use of medication

2.1 Describe person centred ways of administering medicines whilst adhering to administration instructions

In this section we will think about the most appropriate and person centred ways of supporting people with their medication. A person with dementia may not have the mental capacity to understand why they need to take medication, or understand any risks involved. If we have to take responsibility for the administration of medication, we must be very clear about national and local policies.

Research and investigate

2.1 Medication policies

Find out about the medication policy in your area of work. What is your role in carrying out this policy?

There are different methods of administering medication, including:

- self-administration
- enabling – assistive technology, medidose packs
- routines of the person with dementia
- meeting preferences/needs of the person with dementia – use of alternative formats: tablets, solutions, melt in the mouth pastilles, patches, drops.

People with dementia, particularly in the early stages, will be able to manage most activities of daily living. Choice, respect and self-determination are all essential in maintaining someone's self-esteem and independence. When considering the ways in which a person with dementia manages their own medication, we must work with them to make decisions appropriate to their abilities and needs. It may be necessary to think about the principles of the Mental Capacity Act 2005.

Key terms

The Mental Capacity Act 2005 provides a statutory framework for acting and making decisions on behalf of individuals who lack the mental capacity to do so for themselves. The Act specifies the principles that must be applied by everyone who is working with or caring for adults who lack capacity.

You must therefore consider: 'Does the person with dementia have the capacity to manage their own medication and if not, what is the **least restrictive way of supporting them**.' This means that we must use a person centred approach, ensuring that we only intervene as much as is necessary to **manage risk** effectively.

Self-administration. This is when the person is able to manage their own medication independently. They may need some gentle prompts like a calendar or diary or a support worker reminding them. They will be able to understand the purpose of the medication they are taking and will not rely on other people to give it to them. This should be encouraged whenever possible. It is good practice to monitor this situation, noting any problems that occur so that if necessary, enabling techniques can be used.

Enabling techniques. It may still be possible for a person with dementia to manage their medication with some support. Two practical solutions are Medidose or dossett boxes or automatic medication dispensers.

Automatic medication dispensers are classed as **assistive technology**.

Key terms

Assistive Technology can be defined as 'any device or system that allows an individual to perform a task that they would otherwise be unable to do, or increases the ease and safety with which the task can be performed'.

(Royal Commission on Long Term Care 1999)

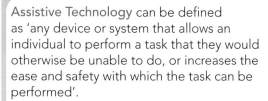

Research and investigate

2.1 **Person centred means of support**

Investigate the types of practical solutions available to support people with their medication. Whose responsibility is it to place the medication in the dispensers?

Although it may not be possible to use such devices in a care home, it is still very important that the dignity of the person with dementia is respected, particularly if the care home has 'drug rounds' as a method of administering medication. Supporting a person with their medication is still a personal intervention. Each person may have a specific way in which they like to take their medication and it is important this is recorded on their care plan. For example one person may prefer to drink from a cup rather than a glass, when swallowing tablets. This attention to person centred detail is important as it can ease the process for all concerned.

If a person declines their medication, you should not force the issue but rather go back after a few minutes. They may have forgotten why they were reluctant. If you are unable to support them, ask a co-worker – remember that it is the person with dementia who must be at the centre of this, not you! If they continue to decline the medication you must record this and inform your supervisor as it may be necessary to re-assess the situation and the person's needs.

Routines are important to all of us. If someone is reluctant to take their medication, think about the routine they may like. Is it possible for the doctor to change the dose or the actual medication so it can be taken at a time or frequency that the person with dementia can cope with?

Think about meeting the preferences/needs of the person with dementia by the use of alternative formats. Tablets, solutions, melt in the mouth pastilles, or patches may be available.

Taking medication can be difficult for any of us and more so for a person with dementia. They may develop physical problems like difficulties in swallowing. If this is the case it may be necessary to consult with a speech and language therapist who is trained to undertake swallowing assessments. Some medication can be prescribed in liquid form, or 'oral dispersible', that is 'melt in the mouth'. If a person is unable to manage oral medication it is possible to use patches, particularly for pain control. Having a person centred approach will assist you in all these decisions – the more you understand about the needs of the person with dementia the more likely you are to find an appropriate way of managing their medication.

2.2 Explain the importance of advocating for an individual with dementia who may be prescribed medication

We have learnt how the different types of medication can affect a person with dementia. All medication carries risks. These include:

- Not seeking medical advice for any adverse effects.
- The person taking the wrong dose (too much or too little).
- Missing doses which will then affect the success of the treatment.
- Medication continuing to be taken when it has been stopped by the doctor.
- Medication being used for the wrong reasons – this might be by the person or by others. If too much or too little medication is deliberately given to a person with dementia this is **physical abuse**.
- Hiding medication in food unless administered under the covert medication policy. Hiding medication unless carried out through the covert medication policy is also classed as physical abuse.

The person with dementia may be unaware of these risks and it is the support worker's duty of care to be mindful of them, to be observant and to report any concerns to the relevant person.

This might be their line manager, the GP or a mental health professional.

A pill in the jam!

There are occasions when although the person with dementia will not comply with medication it is assessed by the doctor that it is vital the person takes this medication on a regular basis. If this is the case a decision to give medication covertly might be agreed.

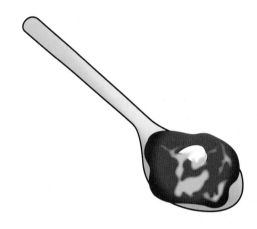

Figure 7.5 'A pill in the jam'.

> ### Key terms
>
> Covert medication is the act of concealing medication a person's food or drink.

This is a decision that must only be taken if it is certain the person always lacks the capacity to understand the consequences of not taking the medication. Mental health practitioners must work within the spirit of the Mental Capacity Act and there may also be occasions when it is more appropriate to treat someone under Section 3 of the Mental Health Act 2007. This means that someone can be detained in hospital to be treated.

The decision to give covert medication must be clearly documented and a full discussion must take place with the person's family or appointed advocate. A care plan must be written explaining why this action has been taken, who made the decision and how the medication will be disguised and when the situation will be reviewed. Before this is done the pharmacist should be consulted about the best way of administering the medication as not all tablets can be crushed, for example. All other forms of medication (patches, dispersible tablets, etc.) should have been considered before the care plan is put in place.

Once the care plan is in place the person with dementia should still be offered the medication overtly (without hiding it). If they continue to decline then the care plan would take effect and this must be recorded to avoid any suspicion of mismanagement of medicines.

Further resources

'Efficacy of treating pain to reduce behavioural disturbances in residents of nursing homes with dementia.' Pub. BMJ 2011 343:d4065doi 10.1136/bmj.d4065

'The use of anti-psychotic medication for people with dementia: Time for action'

(Professor Sube Banerjee, Dept. of Health 2009)

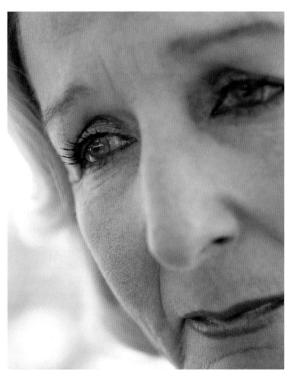

Figure 7.6 How can we help?

Case Study

 Alice

Read the case study and answer the questions. It might be helpful to discuss this with a colleague and your manager.

Alice lives in a care home. She has Alzheimer's disease and arthritis in her knees. Her medication includes Aricept and Paracetamol. She also takes three other types of medication. She used to be a nurse so likes to be busy, often walking about for most of the day. Alice has difficulty with verbal communication. She gets on particularly well with a care worker called Sam.

Lately Alice has become more agitated and upset. She will cry inconsolably and has lately refused to take her medication, often either spitting it out or pushing the care worker away. She is walking more and more slowly. One care worker has been heard to say that

Alice is aggressive and difficult and needs something 'stronger' to calm her down – she might even need to go to hospital as she is such a nuisance and can't be managed.

1) What issues do you need to consider with Alice's medication?

2) Why do you think she is more agitated?

3) How could you find out more about how Alice is feeling?

4) What role could Sam play in this?

5) What are the issues raised by the other care worker – how could these be addressed?

6) What is the home manager's role in this situation?

7) Which other professionals could help you?

8) Write a person centred care plan for Alice, with all your information and conclusions.

Assessment Summary DEM 305

Reading this unit and completing the activities will have provided you with knowledge, understanding and skills required to understand the administration of medication to individuals with dementia using a person centred approach.

To achieve the unit, your assessor will require you to:

Learning Outcomes	Assessment Criteria
1 Understand the common medications available to and appropriate for, individuals with dementia	(1.1) Outline the most common medications used to treat symptoms of dementia See evidence activity 1.1, page 188
	(1.2) Describe how commonly used medications affect individuals with dementia See research and investigate activity 1.2, page 189
	(1.3) Explain the risks and benefits of anti-psychotic medication for individuals with dementia See evidence activity 1.3, page 191
	(1.4) Explain the importance of recording and reporting side effects/adverse reactions to medication. See time to reflect 1.4, page 191
	(1.5) Describe how 'as required' (PRN) medication can be used to support individuals with dementia who may be in pain See research and investigate activity 1.5, page 193
2 Understand how to provide person centred care to individuals with dementia through appropriate and effective use of medication	(2.1) Describe person centred ways of administering medicines whilst adhering to administration instructions See research and investigate activities 2.1, pages 193 and 194
	(2.2) Explain the importance of advocating for an individual with dementia who may be prescribed medication See case study 2.2, page 196

References

Alzheimer's Society (2007) *Out of the Shadows*. Alzheimer's Society, alzheimers.org.uk/outoftheshadows

Banerjee, S (2009) *The use of antipsychotic medicine for people with dementia: Time for action*. Department of Health, http://www.dh.gov.uk/prod_consum_dh/groups/dh_digitalassets/documents/digitalasset/dh_108302.pdf

Bryden, C (2005) *Dancing With Dementia: My Story of Living Positively With Dementia*. Jessica Kingsley Publishers

Care Quality Commission (2011) *Essential Standards of Quality and Safety*. Care Quality Commission, www.cqc.org.uk/standards

Department of Health (2001) *Valuing People: A New Strategy for Learning Disability for the 21st Century*. Department of Health: www.dh.gov.uk

Department of Health (2008) *End of Life Care Strategy – Promoting High Quality Care for all Adults at the end of life*. Department of Health: www.dh.gov.uk

Department of Health (2008) *Introduction to Personalisation*. Department of Health

Department of Health (2009) *Living Well With Dementia: a National Dementia Strategy*. Department of Health: www.dh.gov.uk

Kitwood, T (1997) *Dementia Reconsidered: The Person Comes First*. Open University Press

Stokes, G (2000) *Challenging Behaviour in Dementia: A Person-centred Approach*. Speechmark Publishing

Index